Anti-Aging
HACKS

200+ Ways to Feel—and Look—Younger

KAREN ASP

ADAMS MEDIA

NEW YORK   LONDON   TORONTO   SYDNEY   NEW DELHI

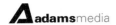
adamsmedia

Adams Media
An Imprint of Simon & Schuster, Inc.
57 Littlefield Street
Avon, Massachusetts 02322

First Adams Media trade paperback edition January 2019

ADAMS MEDIA and colophon are trademarks of Simon & Schuster.

For information about special discounts for bulk purchases, please contact Simon & Schuster Special Sales at 1-866-506-1949 or business@simonandschuster.com.

The Simon & Schuster Speakers Bureau can bring authors to your live event. For more information or to book an event contact the Simon & Schuster Speakers Bureau at 1-866-248-3049 or visit our website at www.simonspeakers.com.

Interior design by Erin Alexander

Manufactured in the United States of America

10 9 8 7 6 5 4 3 2 1

Library of Congress Cataloging-in-Publication Data
Names: Asp, Karen, author.
Title: Anti-aging hacks / Karen Asp.
Description: Avon, Massachusetts: Adams Media, 2019.
Series: Hacks.
Identifiers: LCCN 2018038266 (print) | LCCN 2018040764 (ebook) | ISBN 9781507209561 (pb) | ISBN 9781507209578 (ebook)
Subjects: LCSH: Aging. | Aging--Physiological aspects. | Older people--Health and hygiene. | Self-care, Health. | BISAC: HEALTH & FITNESS / Healthy Living. | SELF-HELP / Aging.
Classification: LCC QP86 (ebook) | LCC QP86 .A87 2019 (print) | DDC 613.2--dc23
LC record available at https://urldefense.proofpoint.com/v2/url?u=https-3A__lccn.loc.
gov_2018038266&d=DwIFAg&c=jGUuvAdBXp_VqQ6t0yah2g&r=eLFfdQgpHVW0iSAzG8F-
WtSjrFvCD9jGMJBHtzyExXhmHvwB7sjMCnFuKz95Uyqa&m=CzO4qAO-FkYqA-AcGjton2sfO
kKDJbweLsLbbp2QLeg&s=D_qIzv1m9I6dR4Hx8tqVfzitKQZmdoRPUSTfP6xJfbY&e=

ISBN 978-1-5072-0956-1
ISBN 978-1-5072-0957-8 (ebook)

CONTENTS

Introduction..6

001. Eat Fruit Instead of Processed Sugar................7
002. Chase an Alcoholic Drink with Water.................8
003. Say Thanks Before You Close Your Eyes.............9
004. Rethink Your Window View.........................10
005. Personalize Your Exfoliation Routine.............11
006. Move Around While You Watch TV...................12
007. Know Your TMAO...................................13
008. Keep Your Waistline in Line.......................14
009. Wear Large Sunglasses (Even on Cloudy Days).......................................15
010. Get a Grip.......................................16
011. Swap Soda for Sparkling Water.....................17
012. Stop Slouching...................................18
013. Bring Your Phone to Eye Level to Fight Tech Neck.....................................19
014. Avoid Pollution During Outdoor Activities.........20
015. Take the Sitting-Rising Test.......................21
016. Trade Fries for a Smarter Side.....................22
017. Slather on Sunscreen 365 Days a Year.............23
018. Stop Sucking Straws...............................24
019. Lighten Stretch Marks Naturally...................25
020. Combat Wrinkles with Retinol......................26
021. Think of Exercise in Ten-Minute Chunks.............27
022. Become a Morning Person..........................28
023. Tint Your Car Windows............................29
024. Rethink a Summer Tan............................30
025. Switch to Non-Dairy Milk.........................31
026. Boost Your Intake of Leafy Greens..................32
027. Slip Into a Sauna................................33
028. Adopt a Dog....................................34
029. Make Your Own Natural Hair Volumizer............35
030. Shun Secondhand Smoke..........................36
031. Roll Up Your Car Windows to Avoid Pollution...37
032. Replace One Meat-Based Meal a Week with a Bean-Based One.....................38
033. Minimize Eyelid Wrinkles with Coconut Oil......39
034. Do Facial Exercises..............................40
035. Lower Your "Fitness Age".........................41
036. Floss Daily.....................................42
037. Read a Book for Thirty Minutes a Day.............43
038. Assess Your Heart Health........................44

039. Whiten Your Teeth...............................45
040. Eat More Vegetarian Meals.......................46
041. Sleep on a Satin or Silk Pillowcase.................47
042. Load Up on Lycopene.............................48
043. Get to Know Your Lp(a)..........................49
044. Find a Feline Friend.............................50
045. Get a Natural Glow from Smoothies................51
046. Count Your Alcoholic Drinks......................52
047. Add Sun Protection to Your Flight Plan............53
048. Catch a Concert................................54
049. Check Sunscreen Expiration Dates................55
050. Enjoy an Avocado a Day..........................56
051. Breathe Away Stress.............................57
052. Turn Down the Heat and Turn Up the Humidifier................................58
053. Drink Coffee....................................59
054. Ditch Your Car for One Trip a Week...............60
055. Shorten Your Shower.............................61
056. Embrace Oats...................................62
057. Practice Yoga Regularly..........................63
058. Dress in a Wardrobe That Fits and Flatters You...................................64
059. Shake the Salt Habit.............................65
060. Smear SPF on Your Lips..........................66
061. Use a Skin Serum with Ferulic Acid...............67
062. Eat Strawberries to Have Better Skin..............68
063. Choose Safer Food Storage Containers............69
064. Wash Your Face Before Bed.......................70
065. Eat the Rainbow................................71
066. Take a Yearly Vacay............................72
067. Green Your Grilling..............................73
068. Craft a Life Purpose Statement to Improve Well-Being...............................74
069. Fast for Twelve to Fourteen Hours a Day.........75
070. Don't Sit for More Than Thirty Minutes at a Time................................76
071. Embrace Meatless Mondays........................77
072. Get Bronzed Sans the Sun........................78
073. Keep Your Hands Looking Young..................79
074. Eat Smaller Fish................................80
075. Enjoy a Roll in the Hay..........................81
076. Eat the Daily Dozen.............................82

077. Re-Establish Good Sleep Habits 83
078. Get Out of Bed If You Can't Sleep 84
079. Pump Some Iron 85
080. Boost Your Fiber Intake with a
     Salad Appetizer 86
081. Eat Your Biggest Meal First 87
082. Set Up a Sleep Sanctuary 88
083. Seek Help for Depression 89
084. HIIT It 90
085. Set a Daily Step Goal 91
086. Use AGE-less Cooking Techniques 92
087. Spice Up Your Food 93
088. Say No Thanks to Receipts 94
089. Drink Green Tea for Supple Skin 95
090. Use Your Face Lotion on Your Arms 96
091. C the Change 97
092. Make a Homemade Lavender Skin Mister 98
093. Volunteer Regularly 99
094. Have Faith 100
095. Consider Fillers 101
096. Be Skin Savvy When Inserting Contacts 102
097. Sleep on Your Back 103
098. Beware Runner's Face 104
099. Walk Faster 105
100. Stay in Healthy BMI Range 106
101. Boost Your Fruit and Vegetable Intake 107
102. Give the Skin Around Your Eyes TLC 108
103. Add Contrast to Your Face 109
104. Meditate for One Minute a Day 110
105. Eat More Blueberries 111
106. Cherish At Least Five Friends 112
107. Replace Meat with Mushrooms 113
108. Enjoy the Morning Light 114
109. Go Nuts 115
110. Dip Into Some Hummus 116
111. Try DIY Solutions for Age Spots 117
112. Maintain Top Dental Health 118
113. Improve Your Balance 119
114. Moisturize with Shea Butter 120
115. Switch to Avocado Butter 121
116. Avoid Canned Foods 122
117. Add Soy to Your Diet 123
118. Hang with Healthy Folks 124
119. Quit Squinting 125
120. Meet Your Magnesium Needs 126

121. Make Your Own Natural Cleaners 127
122. Don't Get Bagged Down 128
123. Soothe Dry Eyes 129
124. Reapply Sunscreen Every Two Hours 130
125. Minimize Crow's-Feet with Soy Milk 131
126. Adopt a "Low-Risk" Lifestyle 132
127. Treat Adult Acne Naturally 133
128. Sing! 134
129. Embrace Hugging 135
130. Look Surprised 136
131. Fight Age Spots with Turmeric 137
132. Tone Flabby Arms 138
133. Apply Cabbage to Varicose Veins 139
134. Relieve Aching Muscles with a Foam Roller ...140
135. Detox Your Skincare Products 141
136. Get Married 142
137. Choose a Flattering Haircut 143
138. Spend Time in Green Spaces Every Day 144
139. Use Tape to Ward Off Brow Wrinkles 145
140. Avoid CFL Lightbulbs 146
141. Connect with Your Community 147
142. Drink Plenty of Water 148
143. Put Blue Light to Bed 149
144. Keep Turkey Neck at Bay with Exercises 150
145. Wrinkle-Proof Your Chest 151
146. Protect Your Hearing 152
147. Pass on Processed Foods 153
148. Eat Prunes for Strong Bones 154
149. Take a Cat Nap 155
150. Trade Potato Chips for Kale Chips 156
151. Keep Track of Your Flexibility 157
152. Banish Brown Spots 158
153. Buy Organic 159
154. Take Makeup Off Before Bed 160
155. Apply a Face Mask at Home 161
156. Consider Collagen Supplements 162
157. Check Out a Sunscreen Pill 163
158. Go Forest Bathing 164
159. Be a Daily Instagrammer 165
160. Eat Almonds to Avoid Gray Hair 166
161. Add Shine to Dulling Hair 167
162. Test for D-ficiency 168
163. Boost Your Lashes, Naturally 169
164. Stop Wearing Your Cell Phone 170
165. Assess Your Gut Health 171

166. Hop on the CoQ10 Bandwagon for Smooth Skin 172
167. Watch Your Tablet Properly 173
168. Reduce Eye Puffiness.....................174
169. Shut Off Your Router at Night.............175
170. Rid Your Mouth of Bacteria with Coconut Oil...176
171. Moisturize Your Skin.....................177
172. Ditch Plastic Bottles.....................178
173. Avoid Muffin Top with Higher-Waisted Pants..179
174. Dry-Brush Your Skin......................180
175. Fight Thigh Dimples with Strength Training ...181
176. Spit Out the Gum 182
177. Take the Stairs.........................183
178. Write in a Worry Journal 184
179. Care for Your Nails......................185
180. Avoid Metal Aviator Frames..............186
181. Watch What You Eat to Avoid Acne.................187
182. Ferment Your Foods 188
183. Don't Squint at Your Computer Screen 189
184. Forgive...............................190
185. Use an Oatmeal Mask on Oily Skin...........191
186. Go Nuts! (Brazilian, That Is) 192
187. Lower Your Resting Heart Rate 193
188. Laugh Every Day 194
189. Avoid Crepey Skin 195
190. Minimize Spider Veins with Warm Coconut Oil...................196
191. Exfoliate Your Hands.....................197
192. Soften Dry Feet.........................198
193. Reverse Yellowing Fingernails 199
194. Treat Yellowing Toenails 200
195. Let Lavender Lull You to Sleep..............201
196. Grease Up Dry Skin on Your Joints 202
197. Stop Using Harsh Soaps 203
198. Weigh Yourself Daily.....................204
199. Try Argan Oil on Your Face...............205
200. Make Your Own Foot Scrub 206
201. Have ED Checked Out 207
202. Exfoliate Your Lips......................208
203. Only Rub Your Eyes Gently................209
204. Don't Rest Your Head in Your Hands...........210
205. Grow Plants in Your Home 211
206. Give Your Brows a Boost 212
207. Add Sea Plants to Your Skincare Regimen 213
208. Pamper Thinning Tresses 214
209. Draw a Beer Bath to Brighten Skin................215

210. Limit Screen Time.......................216
211. Give Up Modern Conveniences Once in a While 217
212. Avoid Exercise-Induced Breast Sagging........218
213. Get Rid of Unwanted Facial Hair....................219
214. Apply Moisturizer with Upward, Circular Motions 220
215. Sip Red Wine 221
216. Know Your Bra Size 222
217. Try Matcha............................223
218. Minimize Knee Wrinkles..................224
219. Soak in a Salt Bath......................225
220. Don't Overeat 226
221. Stop Using Vegetable Oils 227
222. Tighten Your Pores with Artichokes................228
223. Add Seeds to Your Diet 229
224. Measure Your Mile Speed 230
225. Sip Your Greens........................231
225. Embrace Probiotics......................232
227. Jump!................................233
228. Soften Elbow Skin 234
229. Lighten Your Workload 235
230. Use a Headset When Talking on Your Cell Phone 236
231. Filter Your Water 237
232. Say Goodbye to Heavy Earrings 238
233. Darken Your Brows......................239
234. Don't Yo-Yo Diet.......................240
235. Eat Breakfast..........................241
236. Make a Face Mask from Coffee Grounds 242
237. Look at Your Cereal's Nutritional Facts 243
238. Tan with Turmeric 244
239. Stand Up..............................245
240. Moisturize More Often When You're on Medications....................246
241. Enjoy Dark Chocolate in the Morning 247
242. Boost Your Intake of Omega-3s.................248
243. Ventilate Your House.....................249
244. Give Yourself an At-Home Facial Steam 250
245. Don't Skip Meals 251
246. Moisturize with Olive Oil in a Pinch..............252
247. Eat Some Seaweed 253
248. Celebrate Your Age 254

INTRODUCTION

Wrinkles, sunspots, aches, and ailments—aging is not something most people look forward to. But do you need to just resign yourself to losing your looks and your health? No! Forget what you think you know about aging, and instead approach your future with positive energy, healthy choices, and a celebration of all that your body does.

Through the 200+ hacks in this book, you'll learn how to change old habits that aren't serving you well, and adopt simple tricks and tips all in the name of keeping your health—and your looks—intact. You'll discover how to maintain a more youthful appearance, increase your energy, improve your health, prevent chronic disease, have a more positive outlook, and find more joy in life. Best of all, these ideas are easy to implement, simple to fit into your daily lifestyle, and produce real results! For example:

- Have a stiff neck from hunching over? Flip to hack #12 to learn how to adjust your posture.
- Do your hands look older than your years? Try the ideas in hack #73 to improve their appearance.
- What is your RHR and why is it an important measure of your fitness level? Read hack #187 to find out.
- Vegetable, canola, olive...which oil is considered healthy? Hack #221 boils it down and shows you how to cook without any oils!

Whether you're in your twenties or eighties or somewhere in between, these easy hacks will have you looking and feeling younger!

EAT FRUIT INSTEAD OF PROCESSED SUGAR

Want to slow the aging process? Quit indulging your sweet tooth with food-like products that contain added sugar and instead, reach for nature's candy to quell your sweet desires.

Added or processed sugar (not the natural kind from fruits and vegetables) attaches to proteins and fats in your body to create harmful molecules called advanced glycation end products (AGEs). AGEs interfere with collagen and elastin, two compounds your skin needs to maintain its youthful appearance. Collagen is crucial for your skin's structural support, while elastin is responsible for your skin's resilience. Because AGEs prevent efficient collagen repair, you wind up with premature skin aging, and when elastin is affected, your skin elasticity is reduced. The end result? You look older.

Plus, sweets can pack on pounds, and high-sugar diets have been linked to diseases like cancer and Alzheimer's. Look for added sugars, which are in 74 percent of packaged goods sold in grocery stores. Sugar has at least sixty-one different names, including agave nectar, cane juice, caramel, corn syrup, dextrose (and anything else ending in "ose"), molasses, and rice syrup. The American Heart Association recommends limiting daily added sugar intake to six teaspoons if you're a woman and nine teaspoons if you're a man.

Bottom line: when you stop eating as much sugar, you'll then crave less sugar. How can you cut back your added sugar intake? Whenever you're craving something sweet, reach for fruit instead. Try grapes, strawberries, and pineapple for that extra burst of sweetness. You can also put frozen fruit, like raspberries and mangoes—add a banana for more creaminess—in a food processor and blend until smooth for a frozen dessert treat.

CHASE AN ALCOHOLIC DRINK WITH WATER

Besides the hangover, happy hour comes with another side effect you probably didn't know about: wrinkles. Alcohol is one of the biggest promoters of skin aging because it dehydrates the skin. The more dehydrated your skin is, the more prominent your wrinkles. When you compare the skin of lifelong drinkers to that of teetotalers, those in the latter category look much younger—by as much as ten years, according to some experts.

Plus, while there's some data to indicate that certain alcohol does have benefits, lowering risk of heart disease and aiding brain health, other data suggests otherwise. Negative consequences include brain damage, increased risk of cancer, heart problems, and a shortened lifespan.

With this conflicting data, what's a cocktail lover to do? Start by slugging a glass of water with every drink you have, and then simply drink less to be safe. (And if you're not a cocktail fan, there's no reason to start.) How much is safe to drink? A study funded by the British Heart Foundation (BHF) found that the safe upper limit is five glasses of alcohol (either 3.5 ounces of pure alcohol, just over five 20-ounce pints of 4 percent ABV beer, or five approximately 6-ounce glasses of 13 percent alcohol) per week.

SAY THANKS BEFORE YOU CLOSE YOUR EYES

You don't have to wait until late November to feel thankful. Instead, think of three things you're grateful for right before you close your eyes to go to sleep every night.

Research shows that people who are more grateful have better overall health, sleep better, have less anxiety and depression, and are more satisfied with life. Being grateful also triggers the release of endorphins, known as the "happy hormone." In turn, you'll likely lower your blood pressure and heart attack risk, and all of that combined will no doubt lead to a happier, longer life.

Most people do *want* to practice gratitude, but it's hard to remember every day. So each night while you brush your teeth, get into the habit of thinking of three things that happened during the day that you're grateful for, even if they're as simple as the beautiful design the barista created in your latte this morning or the compliment you received from a coworker.

RETHINK YOUR WINDOW VIEW

Think you're safe from the sun just because you're inside? Not if you're sitting by a window! Ultraviolet (UV) rays can stream through windows, and although most windows block UVB rays, there's a second type, UVA, that easily passes through. That UVA can then cause DNA damage in your skin, accelerating skin aging and even causing skin cancer.

To protect yourself, move away from direct light as much as possible whenever you're indoors, whether at home, in your office, or at a restaurant. It's always good to enjoy natural light—just stay out of its direct path when possible. For instance, if your office desk gets direct sunlight, move your desk away from the path of the sun, and when going out to lunch with friends, opt for tables near windows but not in direct sunlight. Also, wear a broad-spectrum sunscreen with an SPF of 30 or higher every day, and if you do get stuck sitting indoors in sun, throw a sweater or jacket (or even a napkin if it's your legs) on overexposed skin.

PERSONALIZE YOUR EXFOLIATION ROUTINE

Exfoliation isn't something only spas—or women—do. Get into a routine of exfoliating at home, and your skin will look younger and healthier.

The process removes dead skin cells from your skin's outer layer, which can make your skin not only look brighter but also younger by increasing your skin's collagen production. Your skin needs collagen for firmness and structure, and as you age, your collagen production slows. Plus, skin cells don't turn over as quickly as you age, which means dead skin cells hang out even longer on your skin—all the more reason why exfoliating becomes even more important with each birthday.

To exfoliate at home, know your skin type. If your skin is shiny and greasy, you have oily skin. If it's rough, itchy, or flaky, you have dry skin. If it burns or stings after using products, you have sensitive skin. If it's oily in spots but dry in others, you have combination skin. If none of these fit your skin type, you most likely have normal skin. People who have dry or sensitive skin might do best with more mild options like salicylic acid peels. Meanwhile, people with oily skin might choose stronger chemical treatments like a salicylic acid wash or a scrub or brush. Your skin type will also tell you how often you should exfoliate. While once a week should be okay for dry or sensitive skin, people with oily or thick skin might be okay doing it daily.

Just use caution, warns the American Academy of Dermatology. Aggressive types of exfoliation could make acne and rosacea worse and may even increase your skin's dark spots. So do your homework about products you're using, and if necessary, consult with a dermatologist.

MOVE AROUND WHILE YOU WATCH TV

Being a couch potato isn't good for your waistline, your appearance, or your overall health. Here's the kicker about those marathon TV sessions: for every hour of TV you watch after the age of twenty-five, you shave 21.8 minutes off your life, according to a study in the *British Journal of Sports Medicine*. Worse? Watching six hours a day on average throughout life means you'll live 4.8 years fewer than people who watch no TV.

The reason is probably obvious: watching TV is a sedentary activity, which raises the risk of diseases like heart disease and diabetes. Not to mention, of course, that you might also eat junk food (hello, potato chips!) while you watch, even though you're not hungry. Before you know it, you've downed that whole bag of chips, and your pants now fit a lot tighter.

While it would be ideal to ditch the TV completely, it is helpful to commit to moving at least 50 percent of your viewing time to doing something active, whether that's walking on a treadmill, pedaling a bike (even a desk cycle), marching in place, or doing stretches or strength exercises. At the very least, get up and move around every fifteen to twenty minutes or exercise during commercial breaks.

KNOW YOUR TMAO

Do you eat meat regularly? Then you might consider getting your trimethylamine N-oxide (TMAO) checked.

What on earth is trimethylamine N-oxide? TMAO is a compound your liver makes. When you consume red meat, egg yolks, and dairy products, you're chomping choline. You also get L-carnitine from red meat and some energy drinks and supplements. Your gut bacteria then digests choline and L-carnitine and produces a compound called trimethylamine (TMA). That's converted by your liver into another compound called TMAO.

If you've got high TMAO levels, you're at greater risk of heart attack, stroke, and death. Studies from Cleveland Clinic have shown that people with the highest TMAO levels are 2.5 times more at risk for those three conditions, even after adjusting for other risk factors like high blood pressure and diabetes. TMAO not only makes it easier for cholesterol to accumulate in your arteries and form plaque (the root cause of heart disease), it also reduces your body's ability to get rid of LDL (or bad) cholesterol.

A blood test can determine if your TMAO level is high. Currently, Cleveland HeartLab in Ohio is one of the few labs offering it. If your level is high, you can then modify your diet to lower it by limiting or avoiding foods such as full-fat dairy products and butter, red meat, and supplements and energy drinks that contain choline, phosphatidylcholine (lecithin), and/or L-carnitine. Then shift as much as possible to a Mediterranean or plant-only diet, as vegans and vegetarians generally produce little TMAO.

KEEP YOUR WAISTLINE IN LINE

Your waist measurement is a good indicator of whether you're at risk for health issues like high blood pressure, high cholesterol, and diabetes, all of which can increase your risk of heart disease and stroke. Obesity is also a separate risk factor for heart disease, and while the scale will tell you how much you weigh, it won't tell you if you have dangerous visceral fat around your abdomen.

Visceral fat lies among your organs—it's not the kind you feel when you try to "pinch an inch"—and it's problematic because it releases fatty acids, inflammatory markers, and hormones that damage your health. Measuring your waist circumference is one of the easiest ways to tell if your abdominal fat is jeopardizing your health and, ultimately, your life.

To get an accurate reading, place the tape measure around your natural waist (right above your belly button). Your waist circumference should be less than forty inches if you're a man and less than thirty-five inches if you're a woman, according to the American Heart Association.

WEAR LARGE SUNGLASSES (EVEN ON CLOUDY DAYS)

Sunglasses are like sunscreen for your eyes, so if you want to avoid wrinkling from UV damage, invest in a pair and wear them whenever you're outdoors. Your eyes and the skin around them can be damaged by the same UV rays that cause sunburn on the rest of your body. Eyes that are exposed to UV light can develop cataracts and macular degeneration, both of which affect vision. UV rays can also cause sunburn of the eyelids and eyes, cancers on or around the eyes, red or swollen eyes, and yes, those dreaded wrinkles.

That's why it's important to wear UV-protective sunglasses (ask your optometrist if you're not sure if yours are UV-protective) whenever you're outside, even on cloudy days. A whopping 31 percent of solar radiation can still pass through clouds and damage eyes. Also, remember that sand, water, and snow can reflect UV rays—at a beach, sand or water can reflect up to 25 percent, while snow-covered surfaces can reflect up to 80 percent—and increase your exposure.

Check that any glasses you wear have 99 to 100 percent UV protection. For more protection around your eyes, the Skin Cancer Foundation recommends larger frames (they cover more of your face) and wraparound styles so you get more peripheral shade.

GET A GRIP

Your grip could help predict whether major diseases, even an early death, are looming in your future, which is why strengthening it should be a priority. A study from the University of Glasgow measured grip strength in more than 500,000 participants aged forty to sixty-nine and examined the link between grip strength and various health issues. Lower grip strength was associated with higher incidence of adverse health outcomes like cancer, and also predicted the risk of death and heart disease even more strongly than physical activity and systolic blood pressure. On the flip side, higher grip strength was linked with a reduced risk of all causes of death.

So how do you build grip strength, which declines as you age? Try these exercises:

1. **Fingertip push-ups:** Get in push-up position on the floor, with your wrists under your shoulders and your legs extended behind so your body is in one long line (drop to your knees if this position is too tough). Tent your fingers so that your fingertips are the only part of your hand touching the floor and perform push-ups using only your fingers.

2. **Farmer's walk with weights:** Stand with your feet together, holding one kettlebell or weighted plate in each hand. Keep your four fingers on one side of the handle/plate and your thumb on the other. Walk approximately thirty feet and turn around, walking back to where you started. Place the weights on the floor and rest for up to a minute, then repeat several times.

SWAP SODA FOR SPARKLING WATER

You know you need to cut out as much processed sugar from your diet as possible, but where should you start? If there's one sugar product you should avoid at all costs, it's soda. What's one easy way to get the same fizz without the negative skin and health consequences? Sparkling water.

Just one can of soda contains ten teaspoons of sugar, and if you don't cut calories elsewhere, you could gain up to 5 pounds in a year just from drinking soda. But that's not all. That soda also causes your skin to sag, because the fructose in soda stimulates a process in your body called glycation. Glycation can break down your skin's collagen and elastin, leaving you with less elasticity in your skin, sagging skin, and wrinkles. Soda can even cause inflammation that makes acne, eczema, and red skin worse.

Soda also ages you internally. That one can of sugary soda a day could age your immune cells by almost two years, according to a study in the *American Journal of Public Health*. Drink a twenty-ounce soda every day and you've just internally aged an additional 4.6 years. People who drink more sugary drinks like soda tend to have shorter telomeres, which are the caps at the end of your chromosomes. Many experts equate them with that cap at the end of your shoestrings. Without that cap, your shoelaces would unravel. Same with your body: shorter telomeres have been linked to shorter lifespans and increased risk of heart disease, diabetes, cancer, even added stress.

So say sayonara to soda and get a sparkling water maker. Then flavor it with whatever fruits and veggies you love most.

STOP SLOUCHING

Mom had it right: sitting up straight really does pay off. Good posture can make you look thinner (by as much as 5 pounds), and can also help you age better. Posture is actually crucial to everything you do—from breathing and digestion to concentration and circulation. Plus, having better posture just makes you feel better. According to a study from *Biofeedback*, slouching increases helpless, hopeless, powerless, and depressive thoughts. Meanwhile, when you walk tall or stand proud, your mood improves and you not only feel younger, you also look younger.

To improve your posture, try to remember these tips. When standing, make sure your knees are slightly bent, shoulders are pulled back, stomach is tucked in, and your head is level, so your earlobes are in line with your shoulders (avoid pushing your head forward, backward, or to the side). When sitting, keep your feet on the floor (use a footrest if necessary) with a small gap between the back of your knees and front of your seat, knees at or below hip level, shoulders relaxed, and forearms parallel to the ground.

Meanwhile, you can help correct poor posture by doing an exercise called angel wings. Stand with your back to a wall, and your feet about four to six inches away from the wall. Lean back so your back is flat against the wall. Bend your arms into stop signs, with elbows bent at shoulder height, hands facing up, and forearms on the wall. Keeping your back, head, shoulders, and forearms against the wall, slide your arms up the wall as high as you can. Return to start and repeat eight to ten times (or fewer if you get too tired to use the correct form). Rest thirty to sixty seconds and repeat. Do this several times a week.

BRING YOUR PHONE TO EYE LEVEL TO FIGHT TECH NECK

If you use any type of digital device, especially a smartphone, you could have tech (or text) neck and, thus, more fine lines and wrinkles. Hunching over smartphones and other devices may be your default position, but it can cause wrinkles and fine lines to develop around your neck. Plus, you'll develop a slumped-over posture, which will make you look older. The human head generally weighs about 10 to 12 pounds, but research has found that when it's tilted 15 degrees forward, it feels more like 27 pounds. When tilted 60 degrees forward, it can feel like 60 pounds. With each degree that you push your neck forward, the stress on your spine increases by 1 degree, which is why there's been an increase in people reporting neck and upper back pain, even among young people. You don't have to be a doctor to diagnose tech neck; just look in the mirror next time you use one of your digital devices and watch how far forward your neck stretches and how curved your spine becomes. (Or ask a friend to take your picture as you use your device.)

While it's difficult to live without devices, you can prevent tech neck by bringing your phone up to eye level. Also, be conscious of your posture as you're using other devices, especially if you're sitting, and arrange your space so that you can maintain an upright posture while using devices.

AVOID POLLUTION DURING OUTDOOR ACTIVITIES

Polluted air could wreak havoc on your complexion and make you look older. Your skin is one of the most important barriers against pollution, yet exposure to harmful pollutants weakens that barrier, allowing unwanted substances to penetrate the skin and cause premature skin aging, pigmentation spots, and even acne. Research has found that an increase in exposure to soot and particles from traffic was associated with 22 percent more pigment spots on the forehead and 20 percent more on the cheeks. In another study, the number of age spots on cheeks increased by 25 percent with only a small increase in pollution, mostly from traffic.

While it's impossible to completely avoid air pollution—recent data from the World Health Organization suggests that over 90 percent of the world's population is breathing unclean air—you can take steps to prevent your skin from pollution-related damage. For instance, next time you're heading outside for a workout or just walking from point A to point B, choose routes that don't have as much traffic. Also, know that pollution can be worse when the weather is calm and during rush hour, according to the Environmental Protection Agency. Plan outdoor activities around these times or, as a last resort, move these activities, even your workouts, indoors.

TAKE THE SITTING-RISING TEST

Can you sit down on the floor and stand without using your hands? This simple test could tell you how long you will live. The sitting-rising test (SRT) requires that you get down on the floor and back up again with as little support as possible. The test measures balance, flexibility, and muscle strength, all of which you need to live longer.

To do the test, wear comfortable clothing and go barefoot. Start from standing and lower yourself to a cross-legged sitting position. Now stand back up, trying not to use your hands, arms, or knees. Score yourself on a scale of zero to ten:

- If you can sit and stand without any support, you earn an automatic ten.
- If you have to use support, deduct a full point.
- Subtract another half of a point if you lose your balance on the way down or up.

In a study in the *European Journal of Preventive Cardiology* of more than 2,000 men and women aged fifty-one to eighty, people who scored less than eight points on the test were twice as likely to die within the next six years, versus those who scored higher. Worse, folks who scored three or fewer points were more than five times as likely to die within the same period, versus folks who scored above eight points. Overall, each point increase on the scale was associated with a 21 percent improvement in survival. No matter your age, this test can be an interesting gauge of your health. But if you're younger than fifty and struggling with the test, consider it a wake-up call to work on your balance and strength, especially in your core and lower body.

TRADE FRIES FOR A SMARTER SIDE

You already know to avoid fast food. But if you are stuck ordering from a fast food eatery for one reason or another, at least skip the artery-clogging, skin-damaging fries and choose a healthier side.

Fast food, in general, is loaded with calories, which can pack on pounds and affect your appearance. Plus, most fast food is high in disease-promoting components: fat, sodium, and sugar, and low in uber-healthy fiber (which you get from foods like vegetables and whole grains).

That junk food causes inflammation in your body, and the more inflammation you have, the greater your risk of heart disease and diabetes. In other words, if you eat crap, you'll feel like crap. You might even look like it, too, as those fries are nothing but refined carbs (a.k.a., refined sugar), which can clog your pores and increase production of pimples, whiteheads, and blackheads. That sugar also creates molecules called advanced glycation end products, which cause premature aging. Plus, fries are loaded with salt!

It's not just the food that's harmful, but also the packaging. A study from the journal *Environmental Science & Technology Letters* found that about one-third of fast food wrappers contains chemicals called poly-fluorinated substances (PFAS) that help make those packages stain resistant and non-stick. PFAS have been linked to increased risk of cancers, high cholesterol, hormone problems, obesity, and immune suppression.

While it's best to skip fast food altogether, at least stop ordering fries, one of the unhealthiest foods on the planet. One study linked the french fry habit—defined by noshing them at least twice a week—with an early death. Instead, choose healthier sides like salad, fruit, or steamed veggies.

SLATHER ON SUNSCREEN 365 DAYS A YEAR

Sunscreen isn't something you only put on when you're at the beach in the middle of the summer. Instead, it should be as much a part of your daily routine as brushing your teeth, even in winter or on cloudy days. That idea might sound like a marketing ploy by sunscreen companies until you consider this: more people are diagnosed with skin cancer than any other cancer, and by the age of seventy, one in five Americans will develop skin cancer, according to the Skin Cancer Foundation. The sun is also responsible for 90 percent of skin aging, and because sun damage is cumulative— by eighteen, you've only accumulated 23 percent of your lifetime exposure, 47 percent by age forty—sunscreen is a must.

Plus, although the sun's rays are most intense on sunny days, you still need sunscreen when it's cloudy. Up to 80 percent of the sun's rays can penetrate through clouds and damage skin.

To keep your skin looking as young as possible, slather on a broad-spectrum sunscreen of at least an SPF of 30 daily (a moisturizer with SPF counts if you're just heading to the office or store). Be sure to get your hands, neck, face (don't forget your eyelids, which is where 10 percent of skin cancers occur), and chest (where you get the most sun exposure). People who do this experience 24 percent less skin aging than those who don't use it daily. Use at least a shot glass–sized amount for your whole body, or a teaspoon for your face. For guidance on buying sunscreen, check out the Environmental Working Group's annual guide to sunscreens, which you can find at www.ewg.org.

STOP SUCKING STRAWS

Ditching straws has recently become an environmental cause—but did you know that sucking on straws causes wrinkles? The movement your mouth makes when it grasps the straw encourages the breakdown of collagen and elasticity more quickly, both of which your skin requires for support. As a result, you get unnecessary wrinkles and lines that make you look like you've been smoking, even if you haven't! If you only use a straw once in a while, it's no big deal. But if you're sucking your cold brew coffee or water from a straw every day, you're asking for wrinkles.

Vanity aside, there's another reason to ask for no straws wherever you eat: Americans use 500 million straws per day on average, according to The Last Plastic Straw. Those straws pollute the oceans, kill marine animals, and get eaten by fish. So do your skin, and the planet, a favor and stop using straws.

LIGHTEN STRETCH MARKS NATURALLY

Stretch marks develop when your skin either shrinks or stretches—whether through normal aging, weight loss, or pregnancy. Shrinking or stretching causes the elastin and collagen in your skin to be disrupted, which may cause stretch marks to appear. They often appear as red, dark brown, purple, reddish-brown, or pink streaks. As time goes on, they may fade and sink below your skin, which is why you eventually may feel a depression over a mature mark.

These marks are permanent, and although many over-the-counter treatments exist to help diminish them, most are not effective. If you'd like to try to lighten the color of your stretch marks, instead try this easy, make-it-yourself lotion: combine 1 tablespoon powdered turmeric, 2 tablespoons aloe vera, and ½ cup organic coconut oil. Apply as frequently as necessary, storing the mixture in a sealed container in a cool, dark place. Expect to see results in six to eight weeks (unless, of course, you have a medical reason to do so).

COMBAT WRINKLES WITH RETINOL

Kiss wrinkles goodbye when you add retinol to your skincare routine! Retinol is a vitamin A derivative that's been proven to reverse signs of aging, smoothing wrinkles, and reversing damage from the sun. Take, for instance, a study from the *Archives of Dermatology* in which thirty-six men and women aged eighty to ninety-six received a lotion with .4 percent retinol on one arm and a retinol-free lotion on the other arm three times a week for twenty-four weeks. As early as four weeks into the study, fine wrinkles in the retinol-treated skin began to fade. After twenty-four weeks, skin roughness and overall severity of the skin's aging had diminished. Researchers explain that the retinol helped retain water and increase procollagen, a precursor to collagen (which is the skin's main support).

Although you can buy many skin lotions and creams that contain retinol over the counter, check ingredient labels to find one with the strength used in the study (.4 percent). If you're not sure of the strength, contact the manufacturer. And it's never too early to start using retinol, even if you're only in your thirties.

THINK OF EXERCISE IN TEN-MINUTE CHUNKS

The fountain of youth is exercise, which is why you should commit to at least thirty minutes a day. Exercise not only keeps skin looking young, possibly by increasing certain substances called myokines made by working muscles that cause changes in cells, it might even *reverse* skin aging. Researchers gathered twenty-nine men and women aged twenty to eighty-four, half of whom logged at least three hours of moderate or vigorous physical activity every week, while the other half were relatively sedentary, exercising less than an hour a week. They then asked each subject to uncover his/her buttock to look at skin rarely exposed to the sun. The surprise? Those over forty who had been active had skin that looked comparable to somebody in their twenties and thirties. To double-check their findings, researchers asked sedentary individuals sixty-five and older to exercise twice a week for thirty minutes to start, progressing to forty-five minutes. Thanks solely to exercise they, too, experienced changes in skin, making their outer and inner layers look similar to people twenty to forty years old.

Beyond skin health, exercise protects you from biological aging, as people who are the most active tend to have the longest telomeres. Telomeres are protective caps at the ends of your chromosomes that shorten as you age and contribute to the aging process. Studies have found that the most active adults are younger on a cellular level (as shown by measures like telomeres) by nine years compared to their sedentary peers.

Government guidelines recommend at least 150 minutes of moderately intense activity (or seventy-five minutes of vigorous activity, or a combination of the two) every week. That breaks down to thirty minutes five days a week, which you can do in one chunk or several five- or ten-minute chunks throughout the day.

BECOME A MORNING PERSON

You've heard the saying that the early birds get the worm. Turns out, they also live longer. That's the news from a study in the journal *Chronobiology International*, which found that night owls, or those folks who stay up late and have trouble getting up in the morning, have higher rates of psychological and neurological disorders and diabetes than morning larks.

Here's something you may not know: whether you're a night owl or a morning lark often stems from genetics. But your environment plays a role, too, and you can try to become a morning person by exposing yourself to light early in the morning (to wake you up more naturally and quickly) and avoiding lots of light at night (especially from screens). Get things done earlier in the day and be less of an evening person as much as possible. Also, keep regular bedtimes and avoid falling back into the habit of crawling into bed late.

TINT YOUR CAR WINDOWS

Sun exposure might not cross your mind when you get into your car. Yet in recent years, dermatologists in the US have noticed an uptick in sun damage on the left side of people's faces. Blame the UV light pouring through your driver's side window.

There are two types of UV rays that damage skin: UVA and UVB. Glass tends to block UVB rays, and although windshields are typically treated to block UVA, side and rear windows aren't, so UVA can easily penetrate. Studies have even found that individuals who drive frequently have more skin color change and deeper wrinkles on the left side of their face, while other research has shown that the left side of the body, especially the head, neck, arm, and hand, receives up to six times more radiation than the right side.

Protecting yourself starts by applying sunscreen with an SPF of at least 30 on your hands, neck, arms, and face about thirty minutes before stepping into your car, according to the Skin Cancer Foundation. Use at least a teaspoon of sunscreen on your face and check that it contains ingredients that protect against UVA, such as zinc oxide, titanium dioxide, and stabilized avobenzone. You should also wear sunglasses and, if possible, a long-sleeved shirt and pants, even a hat if you have a sunroof. You might also consider avoiding driving midday when the sun's rays are strongest. Another potentially easier strategy? Consider tinting or applying a UV-protective film to your car's windows, which could block 99.9 percent of UV rays. (Some states have laws about window tinting, so check your area's regulations before you tint.)

RETHINK A SUMMER TAN

Even though the message about the dangers of tanning has been well known for years, many people still covet tanned skin. Sound familiar? Know this, though: that tan is actually a sign of skin damage, and every time you tan, you increase your risk of developing skin cancer. Melanoma, which is the second most common form of cancer in women aged fifteen to twenty-nine and kills one person an hour in the US, has been largely attributed to UV exposure from the sun and indoor tanning beds, according to the American Academy of Dermatology. Plus, UV rays age the skin prematurely, causing wrinkles and age spots.

Bottom line: there is no "safe" tan, so practice sun safety as much as possible. If you are outside, especially when the sun is at its peak (generally between 10:00 a.m. and 4:00 p.m.), make sure you're protecting your skin with sunscreen and sun-protective clothes and hats. And of course, seek shade whenever you are outside.

SWITCH TO NON-DAIRY MILK

Got acne issues? How about wrinkles? Bet you didn't realize that dairy could be the culprit! Dairy has such a strong link to acne that a study from the *Journal of the Academy of Nutrition and Dietetics* called it a leading cause (along with high-glycemic foods). Why? Cow's milk contains insulin-like growth factor-1 (IGF-1), which could be one driver of acne. Plus, lactose intolerance, which becomes more common as you age, can worsen acne. Dairy has also been linked to increased skin wrinkling.

What about your health? Consuming dairy products has been linked with greater risk of several cancers, namely prostate, breast, and ovarian cancers, as well as obesity, diabetes, and heart disease. Plus, you're ingesting a load of contaminants—anything from hormones to pesticides—that can affect human health. And that assumption that you need dairy to protect against hip fractures? A *British Medical Journal* study followed over 100,000 Swedish men and women for twenty years, and although high milk intake was associated with greater deaths in men and women, women who drank the most milk suffered the most hip fractures (the finding didn't apply to men).

Fortunately, non-dairy alternatives are easier to find than ever, and they contain many of the same nutrients as dairy products. For non-dairy milk, try soy milk, which is most similar in terms of nutrients and texture to cow's milk. If that doesn't please your palate, there's almond, coconut, flaxseed, hemp, and pea, to name just a few.

BOOST YOUR INTAKE OF LEAFY GREENS

Could a salad a day keep aging away? It's possible.

That's one reason Dr. Michael Greger lists greens as part of his Daily Dozen: foods you should eat every day to live not only a high-quality life but a long one too. The reason? "Dark-green, leafy vegetables are the healthiest foods on the planet," he writes.

Here's why he says that. When Harvard University researchers analyzed numerous food groups, greens were associated with the strongest protection against major chronic diseases, including heart attacks and strokes. For every daily serving of greens you eat, your risk of these two diseases drops by about 20 percent.

Then there are the brain benefits you'll enjoy if you eat lots of greens. Healthy seniors who ate a daily serving of leafy greens (½ cup of cooked or 1 cup of raw greens) had a slower rate of cognitive decline, versus folks who ate little or no greens, according to a study in the journal *Neurology*. Those who ate their daily greens had brains that were about eleven years younger than folks who ate less.

Aim for at least two servings a day of greens, which could include arugula, beet greens, collard greens, mustard greens, and turnip greens, as well as kale, mesclun, spinach, and Swiss chard. One serving is 1 cup of raw greens, or ½ cup of cooked. One note, though: if you're taking warfarin (known as Coumadin), talk with your physician before you start eating more greens, as the vitamin K in the greens can interfere with warfarin's efficacy.

SLIP INTO A SAUNA

Some of the world's longest-living individuals, namely the Finns, visit a sauna almost daily. Not Finnish? Who cares? Just follow their lead.

Saunas have been associated with a variety of health benefits, including reducing the risk of heart disease, sudden cardiac death, hypertension, Alzheimer's disease and dementia, and respiratory diseases. Curious why?

So, too, were University of Eastern Finland researchers who looked specifically at the effects of a thirty-minute sauna bath on 100 individuals. The main finding? Both systolic and diastolic blood pressure decreased. Moreover, systolic blood pressure, which is the upper number in your blood pressure reading, remained lower even thirty minutes after stepping out of the sauna.

Next time you book a trip to the spa, make sure you don't skip the sauna (and yes, it's often done in the buff, so don't be surprised). A little pampering to help you live longer? You couldn't ask for a better prescription.

ADOPT A DOG

If you want to live longer, your anti-aging plan might include adding a dog to your family. When researchers looked at the connection between heart health and being a dog parent among records of over three million Swedes aged forty to eighty, they found that people with dogs live longer and healthier. This study didn't identify why dogs offered this protection against death and heart disease, but other studies have shown that dog parents are more physically active and tend to be more social. Researchers even suggest that being around a dog could have positive effects on the bacteria in your gut microbiome, which rules your health.

Regardless of the mechanism, having a dog can do wonders for your happiness and well-being. Of course, it's not a decision to be taken lightly, as adopting a dog is a serious commitment and requires not only time but also financial resources. If you're ready to take the plunge, follow the adopt-don't-shop message and visit a local shelter or rescue organization. And if you already have a dog, all the more reason to give him or her extra TLC. If it's not possible to adopt a dog, ask if you can spend time with a friend's dog, offer to walk your neighbor's dog if he or she is struggling with lack of time or health woes, or volunteer at a shelter or rescue organization.

MAKE YOUR OWN NATURAL HAIR VOLUMIZER

Your hair not only dulls and turns gray with age, it also thins. What many people don't realize, though, is that you can also lose volume in your hair, and less volume often translates to an older appearance. Not only is the density of your existing hair itself decreasing, it's also thinner when it grows in. Research even suggests that this can start happening in women as young as forty.

Want to counteract these changes? Here's what to do. Skip the urge to buy a pricey, chemical-filled over-the-counter product and instead make your own concoction with natural ingredients like ginger, apple cider vinegar, and lemon juice. The combination cleans your hair of anything that's weighing it down and provides antioxidants to your scalp. In a jar, mix 1 tablespoon powdered ginger, 1 teaspoon lemon juice, ¼ cup apple cider vinegar, and ½ cup cool water. Apply the whole batch of treatment after washing your hair while you're still in the shower. Let it sit for two to four minutes, then rinse it out.

SHUN SECONDHAND SMOKE

Even if you're not a smoker, just being around secondhand smoke can age your skin. Whenever you're around smoke, nicotine enters your skin and increases your risk of premature aging and wrinkling as if you were smoking. Plus, more than 41,000 people die every year from secondhand smoke, according to the American Lung Association.

Unfortunately, even just brief exposures to smoke can trigger a heart attack and cause lung cancer and breathing problems like coughing and shortness of breath. The impacts on children can be just as terrible—lung infections, more severe asthma, and a higher risk of sudden infant death syndrome, bronchitis, pneumonia, and ear infections. And don't forget your furry friends: pets are also at risk for health-related complications from secondhand smoke.

All of this means you have to reduce your exposure to smoke. If you're living with a smoker, be a support for that person to help him or her quit smoking. Then enforce a no-smoking policy in your car and house. And although numerous states have enacted laws that prohibit smoking in offices, restaurants, bars, and other public places, not every place is smoke-free, so at least choose smoke-free restaurants when going out to eat and avoid indoor places that allow smoking.

ROLL UP YOUR CAR WINDOWS TO AVOID POLLUTION

Stuck in traffic? Do your skin a favor and roll up those windows, no matter how nice the day is.

Air pollution is a growing threat to skin health, mainly because it damages elastin and collagen. Those are key building blocks in your skin, and when they're impaired, you can develop classic signs of aging like wrinkles, fine lines, dark spots, and crepey skin.

So how does driving through polluted air hurt you? Get this: one study found that pollution *inside* cars driving through Atlanta's rush hour was two times as high as pollution measured outside. Other studies have found pollution inside cars to be ten times as high as the outside air in stations monitoring pollution nearby. Researchers suggest that people in cars get a high dose of pollutants, either through open windows or vents, because they're so close to the source, namely tailpipe emissions.

The best thing you can do is avoid driving during heavy traffic times, as you'll then have fewer cars to pollute the air around you. If you don't have a choice, though, roll those windows up and close the vents so that the air inside your car is recirculated. Also, if you can avoid driving in the morning, even better, as pollution is worse then since it's just sitting on the ground and tends to be thicker, versus after being stirred up.

REPLACE ONE MEAT-BASED MEAL A WEEK WITH A BEAN-BASED ONE

The world's longest-living folks eat beans daily, and if you want to replicate their success, you'll do the same. These long-living people live in what are often called "Blue Zones." Living to one hundred isn't uncommon in these places, and thanks to work done by researcher Dan Buettner and *National Geographic*, five Blue Zones have been identified: Okinawa, Japan; Loma Linda, California; the Nicoya Peninsula in Costa Rica; the Greek island of Ikaria; and the Ogliastra region of Sardinia, an island in Italy.

While these areas share many characteristics, one that links them is regular consumption of beans. Beans are often the centerpiece of meals in these locations—so much that Blue Zoners often eat 1 cup a day. That act alone could add four years to your life.

Beans also factor into Dr. Michael Greger's Daily Dozen. He's the physician and nutrition researcher who wrote *How Not to Die*, which highlights foods you should eat every day. No surprise that beans are on that list—three servings of them daily.

What's the magic behind them (besides their tendency to cause tooting, which will dissipate the more you eat them)? Beans are packed with fiber and protein, plus biotin for healthier skin. They nurture healthy bacteria in your gut, which you need for proper digestion. Beyond that, they also help prevent cancer, lower heart disease risk, improve blood pressure and blood sugar, and may aid in weight loss. An easy way to add more beans to your life is to swap one meat-based meal a week with a bean-based meal. Do this for a few weeks and then increase to two to three bean-based meals a week.

MINIMIZE EYELID WRINKLES WITH COCONUT OIL

Here's a surprising place to find wrinkles: your eyelids. When you're young, your eyelids stay moist with natural oils produced by your body. Yet as you age, you stop producing as much oil, which leads to dryness and, thus, wrinkles. You're also facing the loss of collagen and elastin as you age, both of which give your skin structure, including the skin on your eyelids. Sun damage can also contribute to wrinkling of the eyelids.

To lessen the effect, apply a little coconut oil to your eyelids daily and massage it in gently in a circular motion. That oil will help keep your skin moist, decreasing wrinkles as a result.

DO FACIAL EXERCISES

You do curls for your biceps, squats for your quadriceps, and crunches for your abdominals. But when was the last time you did exercises for your face?

Surprisingly, doing facial exercises could help you look younger, firm your skin, and give you fuller-looking cheeks. That's what a Northwestern University study revealed after sixteen women aged forty to sixty-five did either a daily or every-other-day facial exercise program from Happy Face Yoga for over twenty weeks. Dermatologists rated their faces at three different times during the study and confirmed that the average patient age appearance decreased, starting at 50.8 years and decreasing to almost 48.1 years at the end, an almost three-year drop in age appearance.

Researchers explain that the exercises enlarged and strengthened the facial muscles, making women's faces look firmer, more toned, and, thus, shaped like the faces of younger women. Your skin loses elasticity as you age, which results in fat pads that lie between your skin and muscles thinning. Credit those pads for giving your face shape. Even worse, as your skin starts to sag, the pads actually diminish in size and slide, resulting in a face that "falls." By increasing the size of the muscles in your face, you're basically giving your skin more stuffing, and firmer muscles make that face look more full again.

Here's one you can do anywhere to lift your cheeks: start by smiling. Now make an "O" with your mouth, folding your upper lip over front teeth. Smile again and place your index fingers lightly on the top part of the cheek, directly under your eyes. Relax your cheeks until they return to normal position. Smile again, using the corners of your mouth to lift up your cheek muscles and focus on pushing those muscles toward your eyes. Repeat ten times.

LOWER YOUR "FITNESS AGE"

You can't lower your real age, but lowering your *fitness* age could be one of your best anti-aging strategies. What is fitness age? It's a way to assess how old your body thinks it is, regardless of your real age. While you used to have to go to a lab to determine this, Swedish researchers developed a calculator so anybody can determine their fitness age. You just have to plug in certain numbers like your waistline measurement, maximum heart rate, exercise frequency and intensity, and your weight. Visit www.worldfitnesslevel.org to find a free quiz you can take in less than ten minutes. Check in every six months or so to see if your number has changed.

That's right—your fitness age isn't set in stone. You can always lower it, and you should, especially if it's either the same as or greater than your real age. If your fitness age is higher than your real age, take that as a sign to act. How can you lower your fitness age? Here are three easy ways: shoot for 10,000 steps a day, vary the intensity of your workouts, and build some muscle strength.

Here's why it's key to lower your fitness age: you'll gain additional years in life—about one to two years, according to some studies—and lower your risk of cancer and heart disease. You'll also improve your quality of life, and you'll be able to do more without getting so fatigued.

FLOSS DAILY

Are you someone who flosses right before you have to see the dentist?

You're not alone. Only 30 percent of Americans floss daily, while about 37 percent admit to flossing less than once a day, and 32 percent say they never floss. Despite these dismal reports, the American Dental Association regards flossing as an essential part of your tooth and gum care plan. That floss can help remove plaque, which can lead to cavities and gum disease, in places your toothbrush can't reach.

There's much more to flossing than just plaque removal, however: daily flossing could add an astonishing 6.4 years to your life! The reason lies in flossing's ability to fight gum diseases, which can create inflammation in your body that ultimately damages your arteries and in the end, your heart. To help you remember to floss, make the floss more visible. Set it right next to your toothbrush to remind you to do it.

READ A BOOK FOR THIRTY MINUTES A DAY

Bookworms, rejoice: reading a book, fiction, in particular, could give you a survival advantage.

That's what a study in the journal *Social Science & Medicine* revealed after researchers examined the reading patterns of 3,635 people who were fifty or older. Overall, book readers (most likely fiction, versus newspapers or magazines) lived almost two years longer than non-readers. Reading as little as thirty minutes a day conferred these benefits.

Why is this true? Researchers suggest that books promote cognitive engagement, which may explain why vocabulary, reasoning, concentration, and critical thinking improve. Books also promote empathy, social perception, and emotional intelligence, all of which lead to overall well-being and happiness.

Here are three tips for sneaking in more reading time: swap a thirty-minute TV show with a reading session, read while exercising (audiobooks are perfect for this use), or carry a book with you 24/7 (that's very easy if you use an ereader app on your phone!) and squeeze in reading time whenever you're stuck waiting.

ASSESS YOUR HEART HEALTH

If you're like most Americans, your heart is at risk for various problems—especially as you age. Between 1991 and 2008, the number of Americans with an ideal heart health score dipped from 8.5 percent to 5.9 percent, according to a study in the *Journal of the American Heart Association*. Blame poorer results on body mass index, blood pressure, blood sugar, and cholesterol tests. Meanwhile, those who maintained ideal heart health during that time frame had a lower risk of heart disease and death.

Ready to check how well you're treating your ticker? See how many of these seven habits you can say you do right now (and no cheating!):

1. Manage blood pressure
2. Control cholesterol
3. Reduce blood sugar
4. Get active
5. Eat better
6. Lose weight
7. Stop smoking

How many did you check off? Only 17 percent of adults can say they meet five or more of these seven, and if you're not among them, it's time to get to work. While the earlier you engage in heart-healthy behaviors, the better, it's never too late to start. For more information about all of these behaviors, visit www.heart.org.

WHITEN YOUR TEETH

Few things make you look older than yellow or gray teeth. That's why one of the easiest things you can do to look not only younger but also more attractive is to whiten your teeth. Surveys have found that having white teeth can make you look five years younger and increase your attractiveness by 20 percent. Other research has found that after people's teeth had been whitened, 58 percent of study participants were more likely to be hired, while 53 percent received larger salary offers. Teeth whitening even goes beyond looks, as people were also viewed to be more confident and outgoing after getting their teeth whitened.

Before you do anything, though, talk with your dentist to see if whitening is an option for you. If you have tooth-colored restorations, it may not be wise to pursue whitening. Also, know that whitening can increase tooth sensitivity, although only temporarily, and gingival inflammation. If your dentist gives the okay, you can look for kits at the dental office or over the counter.

You can also try baking soda. Just mix 1 tablespoon of baking soda with 1 tablespoon of water until it forms a paste. Apply that to your teeth and then brush. Do this only about once a week, as baking soda can strip enamel from your teeth, so you don't want to do it too often.

EAT MORE VEGETARIAN MEALS

When it comes to living longer, vegetarians are leading the pack. Numerous reasons might prompt you to push meat aside and eat more plants—but one of the most compelling might come from a study conducted by Harvard T.H. Chan School of Public Health researchers, who found that roughly one-third of early deaths could be prevented if everybody moved to a plant-based diet. In other words, go veg!

The benefits of eating plants over animals extend beyond just living longer. By eating more plants, you'll lower your risk for numerous chronic diseases, including heart disease, cancer, type 2 diabetes, obesity, and rheumatoid arthritis. In some cases, you might even be able to reverse the progress of some of these diseases. A plant-based diet is the only diet that's been proven not only to reverse but also prevent heart disease.

Plus, by eating more plants, your skin quality will improve. People who switch to a plant-based diet sometimes notice that skin issues like acne and redness immediately clear up. Over time, their complexion improves and their skin tone looks healthier.

And of course, the environment and animals will also benefit.

Need help figuring out how to eat veg? Sign up for the Physicians Committee for Responsible Medicine's 21-Day Vegan Kickstart Program (www.pcrm.org/GetHealthy), which starts every Monday. Or visit sites like www.forksoverknives.com, www.onegreenplanet.org, and https://nutritionstudies.org, all of which are loaded with tips and recipes. And if you want to learn more about plant-based eating, watch one of the many documentaries available on the topic, including *Forks Over Knives*, *What the Health*, *PlantPure Nation*, *Cowspiracy*, *Speciesism*, *The Game Changers*, and *Dominion*.

SLEEP ON A SATIN OR SILK PILLOWCASE

Want to avoid dry skin, which makes you look older? Try this: ditch your cotton pillowcase and sleep on one made from satin or silk.

Even if you're using organic cotton, that pillowcase could still be aging your face. Because cotton absorbs moisture, your pillowcase could be sucking your skin dry as you sleep, causing you to look dehydrated when you wake up. Cotton fabric can also worsen sleep lines, which are permanent creases in your skin that form when you repeatedly press your face into a pillow.

Silk or satin pillowcases, however, won't absorb moisture. Plus, the slippery surface lets your skin glide over it, making it difficult to develop sleep lines.

LOAD UP ON LYCOPENE

Tomato or tomahto? Doesn't matter how you say it, just make sure you eat one—or several—a day. Tomatoes and tomato products like paste and sauce are rich in an antioxidant called lycopene, which could be a salve for your skin, not to mention your whole body. In one study from the *British Journal of Dermatology*, women who ate 5 tablespoons of tomato paste every day for twelve weeks had 33 percent more protection against a sunburn than a control group. You still need sunscreen, though, as the lycopene you eat won't offer 100 percent protection against UV rays. Other studies have found that applying lycopene topically can even help reverse damage from UV exposure and encourage cell renewal. It may help your skin maintain its natural firmness too.

Lycopene's benefits extend beyond the skin. It can also help prevent osteoporosis and cancer, especially prostate cancer. Lycopene in tomato juice has been shown to help women lose body fat too.

Eat at least one serving of lycopene-rich foods daily. When possible, choose cooked (like in tomato paste or sauce) versus raw tomatoes. Lycopene from raw tomatoes isn't absorbed as well by your body. Just make sure you check sodium and sugar levels; if possible, choose low-sodium and no-sugar versions. Not a tomato fan? You can also get lycopene from watermelon, pink guavas, and pink grapefruit.

GET TO KNOW YOUR LP(A)

When it comes to cholesterol, you have probably heard of LDL (a.k.a. "bad" cholesterol), HDL (a.k.a. "good" cholesterol), and triglycerides. But have you heard of lipoprotein(a)? It's also known as Lp-little-a or Lp(a).

Roughly 20 percent of the American population has high levels of Lp(a), defined as greater than 50 mg/dL, but most don't know it, according to the Lipoprotein(a) Foundation. With high Lp(a), you're at significantly higher risk of heart disease and heart attack, peripheral vascular disease, blood clots, and stroke. It's passed down from your parents, and a simple blood test can determine whether yours is high.

Although some insurance companies may not cover the cost of the test, you should get your Lp(a) tested if you or a family member has had a heart attack or stroke at an early age (younger than fifty-five for men, sixty-five for women); if somebody in your family has high Lp(a); if you've had a heart attack or stroke with no other known risk factors like high LDL, diabetes, or obesity; if you have high LDL even if you're taking statins or other cholesterol medications; or if you have familial hypercholesterolaemia, an inherited condition of high LDL cholesterol. If you do have high Lp(a), your doctor will work with you to lower your overall heart disease risk, especially if you haven't changed anything about your habits because your cholesterol levels have always been normal. There's nothing you can do to bring down that Lp(a), but you can lower your overall cholesterol by logging regular exercise, slimming down if you're battling weight issues, not smoking, and eating a plant-strong diet.

FIND A FELINE FRIEND

America may be a dog-loving nation—60.2 million households have a dog versus 47.1 million with a cat—but there's good reason to give cats a fair shake. Simply put, cats can prolong your life.

In a study from the *Journal of Vascular and Interventional Neurology*, researchers found that during a twenty-year period, cat parents were less likely to die of a heart attack or stroke than non-cat folks. Non-cat people had a 40 percent greater risk of death by heart attack and 30 percent higher risk of death from any sort of cardiovascular disease than current or past cat parents. Why? Your kitty will also love hearing the answer: the simple act of petting your cat lowers blood pressure, which is why your heart benefits.

Want to bring home a feline friend? There are wonderful cats in shelters and rescue organizations awaiting their forever homes. You can connect with many of them by searching Petfinder (www.petfinder.com) or checking with local shelters. And if you can't bring a cat into your house, consider volunteering to help care for cats at shelters and rescue organizations.

GET A NATURAL GLOW FROM SMOOTHIES

Forget lotions and potions to make your skin glow. Instead, do what Mom always advised and eat your veggies (and fruits)—because you really are what you eat. A study in *PLOS One* found that eating a diet high in fruits and veggies loaded with carotenoids—think red, orange, and yellow pigments—gave Caucasian women an appealing healthy tint to their skin over a six-week period. They also had a more rosy tone to their skin. A second experiment then proved that those changes were seen as healthy and attractive. Researchers explain that the enhanced skin color may have been the result of polyphenols in fruits and veggies that improved blood flow to the skin.

If you're already eating a diet high in fruits and veggies, your skin is probably already glowing. However, if you're like most Americans, you're falling way short of the recommended amount of fruits and veggies you should be eating. By eating six portions of fruits and veggies each day, you could see a healthier and more attractive skin tone in just six weeks.

One way to sneak in more fruits and veggies? Make a smoothie. Another study in *PLOS One* showed that after four weeks of including a carotenoid-rich fruit and veggie smoothie in their diet, Chinese participants had notable positive changes in their skin color. Try this easy and refreshing smoothie: blend a handful of ice with ½ cup non-dairy milk of your choice, 1 medium green apple (cored), 1 date (chopped), 1 to 2 cups chopped spinach, 1 stalk celery, 1 tablespoon ground flaxseed, and 1 tablespoon nut butter of your choice. Blend until smooth and enjoy this large one-serving snack or have it as part of your meal.

COUNT YOUR ALCOHOLIC DRINKS

Sipping alcohol in moderation might help you age better, especially given that research has revealed that alcohol can help you live past ninety.

That news comes from the 90+ Study from the University of California, Irvine's Institute for Memory Impairments and Neurological Disorders, which studies the effects of daily lifestyle habits on individuals over ninety. Those who drank about two glasses of beer or wine a day were more likely to live longer. Booze even beat out exercise (although note that this doesn't give you permission not to exercise).

And beer lovers, science has also confirmed what you may have already guessed: beer makes you happy. Credit hordenine, a substance in beer, for beer's mood-elevating effect. Of course, happiness leads to increased well-being, which then leads to a longer life.

Just remember that moderation is clearly key, especially given all of the conflicting evidence about alcohol. One way to drink less when you're out with friends? Count your drinks. It sounds a little corny, but researchers found that among sixteen behaviors they studied that might help people drink less, counting drinks showed the most benefit. Try using an app like Drink Less or DrinkControl.

ADD SUN PROTECTION TO YOUR FLIGHT PLAN

You may not think about protecting yourself from UV rays when you're flying, but you should. UV radiation is the number one cause of premature aging of the skin, but it's probably the last thing you think about when you're jumping on a plane. Here's why it matters, though: as you ascend to higher altitudes, your exposure to UV radiation increases. For every 1,000 feet you ascend, UV levels increase by 4 to 5 percent.

For pilots and the cockpit crew, this is especially alarming, considering that spending fifty-six minutes in the cockpit at 30,000 feet is the equivalent of spending twenty minutes in a tanning bed. Levels could be even higher when flying through thick clouds and snow, which reflect UV rays. Airplane windows apparently don't block UVA radiation, which can increase the crews' risk of melanoma.

Granted, you may not spend as much time flying as the flight crews, but that doesn't mean you're not getting some exposure to those rays too.

The logical fix? Apply sunscreen to exposed skin before boarding and cover bare skin with a jacket or sweatshirt, especially if you've scored a window seat (although opt for an aisle seat next time). And don't be afraid to lower that shade, the airline will most likely ask you to do that when you land anyway if you're flying during warmer months.

CATCH A CONCERT

Permission granted to buy tickets to see your favorite musician. If anybody gives you grief, tell them this: you're doing it so you can live longer. Why? Jamming to live tunes may extend your life.

It's no secret that music comes with a myriad of health benefits. Studies have found that it can help you fall asleep faster, lower stress, reduce pain, trigger memories in people with dementia, and even motivate you to exercise longer and harder. It can also boost your longevity because music can nurture feelings of health, happiness, and well-being.

In a study conducted by The O2, a music and entertainment venue in the United Kingdom, people who regularly attended live gigs increased feelings of self-worth and closeness to others by 25 percent and mental stimulation by 75 percent. Just twenty minutes of attending a show boosted overall feelings of well-being by 21 percent (versus only 10 percent for yoga and 7 percent for dog walking). Combining this research with other studies, The O2 concluded that those high levels of well-being lead to an increased lifespan of nine years.

How often should you listen live? According to the study, once every two weeks is best. Rock on!

CHECK SUNSCREEN EXPIRATION DATES

Sunscreen isn't like a fine bottle of wine—age that sunscreen too long, and it'll lose its efficacy, upping the odds that you'll get burned. The solution? Do an annual sunscreen audit and toss any that are too old.

Sunscreen usually has an expiration date printed on its packaging. If you don't see one, write the date you purchased the sunscreen on the bottle, label, or can. Then, at least once a year, check those expiration dates. Sunscreen has a shelf life of about two to three years, according to the Skin Cancer Foundation, so throw away any that are older than that. Also, double-check that you're storing in that sunscreen in a cool place. Heat can cause sunscreen to break down, which might also affect its ability to work correctly.

Truth is, though, if you're using sunscreen daily and applying what you need—a shot glass for your whole body, or a teaspoon for your face— you shouldn't have to worry about expiration dates. That sunscreen will be gone before it even has a chance to age.

ENJOY AN AVOCADO A DAY

There's a reason avocado is called nature's butter: whether you eat it or slather it on your skin, it can make you look younger and boost your health.

Avocados contain a good amount of healthy fats, namely polyunsaturated and monounsaturated fats, which can help prevent moisture loss in your skin. They're also high in vitamin E, which is an antioxidant that could protect your skin cells from free radical damage and even UV rays. The benefits are even more evident when you apply mashed avocado to your skin, as it can hydrate dry skin and protect against moisture loss in the future. One study also found that applying avocado oil before going out in the sun helped prevent sunburn (but that doesn't mean you should skip using a sunscreen).

But why stop with your skin? Eating avocados has also been shown to lower cholesterol. Plus, research indicates that not only do avocado eaters have better diet quality, they also have lower body weight, body mass index (BMI), and waist circumference. Compared with avocado abstainers, avocado lovers weigh 7.5 pounds less on average, have a mean BMI of one unit less, and have 1.2 fewer inches around their waists. Avocado eaters are also 33 percent less likely to be overweight or obese.

Here's a simple recipe for an avocado mask you can make at home: mash an avocado until it turns pasty, add water, and apply it to a cleansed face. After fifteen minutes, rinse with water. Use one to three times a week.

BREATHE AWAY STRESS

No buts about it: stress sucks. So fight back with some calculated breath work.

When you're stressed, your body releases hormones called cortisol and adrenaline. This is called the fight-or-flight response, which is why your heart starts beating faster. Those hormones also constrict blood vessels so blood is diverted away from your extremities and directed to your core. As a result, your blood pressure rises. Once the stressful situation ends, everything should return to normal.

Trouble is, many people live with chronic stress, which means their bodies stay on high alert for long periods of time. That can take a toll on the heart, increasing risk for heart attack. Plus, numerous studies have found that women who are chronically stressed have shorter telomeres than women who find more Zen in life. Shorter telomeres are associated with a shorter life.

By getting that stress under control, you can eradicate these issues and perhaps add years to your life. Take those folks in the Blue Zones (see hack #32): one of their keys to longevity is that they know how to downshift and reduce stress. To combat your stress, know your stress triggers and work to find ways around them. Then every day, do at least one thing you enjoy doing and engage in regular exercise, which can help release tension in your body and make you feel better. One thing that's scientifically shown to reduce stress? Deep breathing, but make it count—literally! Simply count your breaths from one to nine (one count equals an inhale and exhale) as many times as you'd like.

TURN DOWN THE HEAT AND TURN UP THE HUMIDIFIER

Cranking the heat in your house is a natural reaction when it's snowing, blowing, and freezing outside. Yet as your insides are warming up, your skin is drying out. Those high temps can suck the moisture right out of your skin, leading to dry and sometimes inflamed skin, which can accelerate the aging process.

Your skin is made up of 64 percent water, but when the environment becomes drier, your skin's outer layer follows suit, even becoming stiffer. The moisture content of your skin plays a role in the development of wrinkles, especially what some experts call micro-wrinkles, which start at the surface and eventually become deeper, larger, and more visible.

Aim to keep the temperature in your house no higher than 68°F. You might even consider adding a humidifier, which increases the water content in the air in your house and moisturizes your skin. Set it to around 60 percent, which should help rehydrate your skin. (And by the way, if you live in an area with a drier climate, like Denver or Las Vegas, your skin may suffer similar effects, wrinkling more after a certain age. Make sure you're moisturizing and using a humidifier.)

DRINK COFFEE

You may not need another excuse to greet the day with a cuppa joe—64 percent of Americans drink coffee daily, reports the National Coffee Association—but here's another: coffee drinkers may live longer.

Numerous studies support that claim, but one of the most telling comes from the University of Southern California in Los Angeles. The study, published in *Annals of Internal Medicine*, involved more than 215,000 individuals from four different ethnic backgrounds, including African Americans, Japanese Americans, Latinos, and Caucasians. Overall, those who drank a cup of coffee a day (either caffeinated or decaf) had a reduced risk of certain cancers, diabetes, liver disease, and Parkinson's.

Do you drink several cups? Believe it or not, other studies have found similar benefits when people sip three to four cups. The shocker was an even more recent study that found that drinking as much as *eight* cups of coffee a day was beneficial!

Coffee isn't for everybody, though. First, if you don't already drink coffee, don't think you have to start. Also, if you have trouble sleeping, avoid caffeinated coffee later in the day. Caffeine has a half-life of three to five hours, which means that it takes your body that amount of time to eliminate half the caffeine. As a result, you could still have caffeine in your system when you go to bed. If you do drink coffee, though, keep it black, as dumping in sugar and cream can add calories and fat to an almost calorie-free drink. (An eight-ounce cup contains only about two calories.)

DITCH YOUR CAR FOR ONE TRIP A WEEK

Your car might be the most convenient way for you to commute to work (or the coffee shop or gym), but if you care about your health, you'll try to ditch the car once in a while and find a more active way to commute—by bike, foot, or even public transportation.

Commuting to work without a car might not be an easy task if you live in suburban America, where roads aren't always conducive to active commuters, and public transport hardly exists. But it's worth a shot. After all, you could cut your risk of heart disease, stroke, and early death by almost one third. Actively commuting to work can also replace a trip to the gym if you're pressed for time, helping you lose as much body fat as those who do high-intensity exercise.

Riding your bike may be one of the best options for most people, but how do you do it? Follow these simple tips from the League of American Bicyclists:

- Wear a helmet and bright clothing so you're visible
- Find a route via Google Map's bike directions and then ride it on a non-work day so you're not pressed for time and can determine if you like the route
- Carry clothes in a saddlebag versus a backpack
- Bring clothes to work that you can keep there and then change into
- If you don't have a shower at work, check into using showers at an on-site fitness center or at least keep baby wipes in your bag or at work
- Bike at a slower speed in hot weather so you sweat less
- Use hand signals and obey stop signs and traffic lights
- Use headlights in the dark

If commuting via bike just isn't feasible for you, trade another car trip for an active one once a week. Whether it's a bike trip to the library, a walk to school, or a jog to watch a sporting event, you're doing your body and the environment a favor.

SHORTEN YOUR SHOWER

Long, hot showers might seem luxurious, but they're not so good for your skin. Statistics from Home Water Works show that the average shower lasts 8.2 minutes, which is a drain on not only the environment (you're using 17.2 gallons of water) but also your skin's natural oils. Long baths or showers (over ten minutes) increase the loss of these oils, which worsens your skin's dryness and can lead to skin aging. And if the water in that shower is hot, you'll lose even more moisture.

Instead, choose short showers over baths, and keep those showers under five minutes long. If possible, take a "navy shower," where you turn the water on to rinse your body and hair, turn it off to shampoo and wash your body, and then turn it on again to rinse off all the shampoo and soap. And although you don't have to embrace the Nordic spa tradition and plunge into a cold bath, do lower the water temperature so it's warm, not hot. After showering, apply moisturizer over your entire body when your skin's a little damp to help it soak in more.

EMBRACE OATS

Oats may not be as trendy as kale or acai berries, but that's not a good reason not to celebrate this underappreciated superfood daily!

When used on the skin, oats have powerful healing effects. They're known for their skin-soothing properties, which is why they're beneficial for sunburns, rashes, and allergic reactions. Their coarse texture also makes them perfect for removing dead skin cells. Because they're humectants, which means they help retain moisture, they can even help moisturize your skin. And they're packed with eighteen different amino acids, which your skin needs to rebuild tissue and promote healing, so oats can help repair damaged skin.

From a health standpoint, oats are heart-healthy, helping in lowering cholesterol and reducing heart disease risk. They've also been found to lower risk of colon cancer and diabetes, stabilize blood sugar, improve immune function, and improve athletic performance and sleep (some experts recommend eating oats before bed). And yes, oats will keep you full longer, which can lead to changes on the scale.

To reap the skin rewards, make a mask with oats. Mix ¼ cup ground oats with 2 to 3 tablespoons of water, stirring until the mixture is a smooth, spreadable paste. Add more water or oats as necessary to get a good consistency. After washing your face and patting it dry, apply the oats to your face, avoiding your eyes. Wait fifteen to twenty minutes and rinse with warm water.

Then start your day by eating oatmeal. Soak steel-cut oats overnight in non-dairy milk or yogurt if you don't have time to spend cooking them in the morning. Just avoid those single-serving instant-oatmeal packages; they're often laden with sugar.

PRACTICE YOGA REGULARLY

If you want to slow the hands of time, aim to hit your yoga mat at least three times a week.

Ancient yogi texts suggest that a regular yoga practice may delay the aging process, and studies now prove that. In one study published in *Evidence-Based Complementary and Alternative Medicine*, yoga was linked to an increase in two substances, dehydroepiandrosterone sulfate (DHEA-S) and growth hormone (GH). They're known as anti-aging hormones (DHEA-S is sometimes called the youth hormone), but they typically decline with age. Unless, that is, you're doing yoga. Twelve weeks of doing yoga six days a week significantly increased both hormones in middle-aged individuals. Another study in *Oxidative Medicine and Cellular Longevity* showed changes in cellular aging after individuals did twelve weeks of yoga and meditation five days a week for about ninety minutes each time.

Yoga also improves numerous variables associated with aging. You'll build balance, especially when you do poses like Warrior and Tree Pose, which can reduce your risk of falling. Yoga helps fight age-related declines in your flexibility, which can affect your daily functioning. And while it's not like lifting weights, yoga can increase muscular strength to some degree, even helping you build some bone density.

If you're new to yoga, take an introductory class from a qualified instructor so you can learn the poses. You can also do yoga at home through DVDs, free *YouTube* videos, or online streaming sites like www.myyogaworks.com, www.yogaglo.com, or www.yogadownload.com. Aim to practice yoga at least three times a week.

DRESS IN A WARDROBE THAT FITS AND FLATTERS YOU

Forget the facelift. If you believe the results of a British study, it might be time to invest in a new wardrobe instead of plastic surgery.

To see how clothing might affect age, British researchers put the same fifty-five-year-old woman in twelve different outfits and asked the public to guess her age. Guesses ranged from forty-seven to sixty-two years old, and it all depended on the outfit. When the woman wore clothes that were fitted and flattering, people said she looked eight years younger. Yet when she donned big jeans and an oversized shirt, people guessed that she was sixty-two.

Ironically, it was the face that the observers based most of their age assessments on. The frumpier and less fitted the clothes, the older the woman's face looked. Moral of the story? Clothes that truly fit your shape are really worth the effort to find and tailor. Start by thinking about the items in your closet you wear most often and invest in high-quality versions.

SHAKE THE SALT HABIT

Got a thing for salty foods? Besides upping your blood pressure, here's another reason to kick salt out of your diet: it could be making you age faster, outside and in. Eating too much salt essentially dehydrates your internal organs, causing them to "steal" water from your skin. As your skin becomes more dehydrated, fine lines become visible and your facial color dulls.

Salt also ages you on the inside. Telomeres are the protective ends on your chromosomes, and although they naturally shorten with age, a sodium-rich diet can make them shorten faster.

The American Heart Association and the American College of Cardiology recommend limiting sodium intake to no more than 1,500 mg a day, although you'll do better going under 1,000 mg a day. One teaspoon of salt, by the way, contains 2,325 mg.

While you should stop salting foods, it's also important to watch out for high-salt processed and prepared foods. A whopping 40 percent of your daily sodium intake probably comes from only ten foods, according to the Centers for Disease Control and Prevention, and white bread of any sort is a big culprit. Here's the full list: bread and rolls, pizza, sandwiches, cold cuts and cured meats, soups, burritos and tacos, savory snacks (like chips, popcorn, pretzels, snack mixes, and crackers), chicken, cheese, and eggs and omelets. Select low-sodium versions of your favorite foods, remove the salt shaker from your table, and use herbs and spices in lieu of salt to flavor foods.

SMEAR SPF ON YOUR LIPS

You know how harmful UV exposure is, and how it's the number one cause of premature aging. That's why you shouldn't leave your lips out of your sunscreen plan.

Your lips get tons of exposure to the sun every day, which is one reason you can develop skin cancer there. The surprise? Your lower lip actually gets more sunlight than your upper lip, making it twelve times more likely to be damaged by the sun, according to the Skin Cancer Foundation. Plus, lips are thin to begin with, and as you age they get even thinner, thus requiring more moisture. As a result, lips can show the same signs of aging and may even age faster than other skin.

So follow this new rule: apply lip balm, lipstick, or a sunscreen stick with an SPF of at least 15 to your lips every two hours, giving that lower lip a little more attention. Doing this will protect against dehydration and those harmful UV rays.

USE A SKIN SERUM WITH FERULIC ACID

Antioxidants are your skin's best friend, and if your skin hasn't yet met ferulic acid, it's time for a beauty change. Ferulic acid might sound like something scientists developed, but it's actually found in nuts, oranges, and apples. It's a potent antioxidant that works against free radical damage. Those free radicals are molecules that circulate in your body, damaging other molecules, which can result in the breakdown of collagen (and thus, the development of wrinkles) and hyperpigmentation.

On its own, ferulic acid can reverse skin damage from the sun and those classic signs of aging, including fine lines and wrinkles. Yet when combined with other antioxidants like vitamin E or vitamin C, it becomes even more effective.

So how do you use it? Look for a serum with ferulic acid (and other antioxidants) and then apply it to your face every morning before moisturizing and applying sunscreen.

EAT STRAWBERRIES TO HAVE BETTER SKIN

Top that morning oatmeal with strawberries and, surprisingly, your skin will benefit.

When mice were exposed to increasing UV radiation for eight weeks, those that received a topical application of ellagic acid, a compound in strawberries, had less sunburn and wrinkle formation. Ellagic acid prevents inflammation and blocks secretion of enzymes that break down the skin's collagen and cause wrinkles.

Even just eating strawberries could help prevent aging. Strawberries also come packed with skin-healthy nutrition, especially vitamin C, which your skin needs to make collagen. In 1 cup of strawberries, you'll get 96 milligrams (mg) of vitamin C, which more than covers the recommended 90 mg daily value. Plus, eat one serving a day—eight strawberries, to be exact—and you may improve heart health, help manage diabetes, support brain health, and reduce the risk of some cancers, according to the California Strawberry Commission.

If possible, choose organic strawberries. If you can't find or afford organic, this shouldn't stop you from buying strawberries, but it's worth checking into, as strawberries can be loaded with pesticides. According to the Environmental Working Group's 2018 Shopper's Guide to Pesticides in Produce, strawberries have the most contamination from pesticides.

CHOOSE SAFER FOOD STORAGE CONTAINERS

Plastic food containers are ubiquitous and are really handy when you want to transport healthy snacks somewhere. But some plastics contain a chemical called bisphenol A (BPA). Although the FDA has largely ignored studies on BPA and considers it safe, BPA is a known endocrine disruptor and has been shown to affect human health, especially in reproductive disorders, heart disease, body weight issues, and breast and prostate cancers. That's why many companies have replaced BPA with bisphenol S (BPS), but unfortunately, BPS may be even more toxic than BPA, as BPS could lead to conditions like diabetes, obesity, asthma, birth defects, and cancer.

If possible, eliminate all plastic from your kitchen and pantry (think of where you store things like raisins, oats, and dry beans) and instead use glass, Pyrex, or stainless steel. If you can't afford to make the switch yet, at least check the number in the triangle on the bottom of your plastic containers. If they have a number two, four, or five, they're generally recognized as safe for food and drink. However, toss (or recycle, if available in your area) those with the number three, six, or seven, as they're considered high-risk.

Another tip: never put plastics in the microwave or dishwasher, as heat can increase the amount of plastic that leaches into your food, and always dispose of any plastic containers that are scratched, cloudy, or badly worn.

WASH YOUR FACE BEFORE BED

As simple as this sounds, washing your face, especially every night before bed, can prevent aging and other skin woes. During a day's time, lots of gunk can gather on your face. Along with any lotions, creams, or makeup you've put on in the morning, your face picks up dust, dirt, pollen, and cigarette smoke, which can damage the skin, leading to wrinkles and sagging. Later, when you're asleep, bacteria and unwanted oil build on your skin, and if none of this pollution is removed, your skin could suffer.

Know your skin type so you can choose the right cleanser. For example, if you have eczema, avoid cleansers with high amounts of benzoyl peroxide, which can irritate and dry out your skin. For most people, it's best to use a gentle, non-abrasive, alcohol-free cleanser versus just water or water and hand or body soap. Water alone isn't enough to do the job, and hand or body soap could irritate facial skin.

First, wet your face with lukewarm water and use your fingers to apply the cleanser, avoiding the urge to scrub. (And don't use washcloths or mesh sponges, as they can irritate skin.) Rinse with lukewarm water and pat dry with a soft towel.

Aim to wash your face twice a day, once after getting up and again before going to bed. Also, if you've sweated heavily, give that face a quick rinse, as sweat can irritate the skin, especially if you've been wearing sunglasses, a hat, or a helmet. If you can't commit to twice-daily face washes, the before-bed wash should be your main priority.

EAT THE RAINBOW

Meeting your daily suggested intake of fruits and veggies becomes a lot more fun when you plan it around the colors of the rainbow. Each color of produce offers different nutrients, and the more colors you eat, the wider the variety of nutrients you'll be consuming. You'll then gain protection from chronic disease and illnesses, including declining vision, colds and the flu, weight issues, heart disease, diabetes, cancers, and more.

With credit to the Food Revolution Summit, here are the benefits of each color and examples of each:

Red Produce

- Main benefits: Helps fight cancer, reduces risk of diabetes and heart disease, and improves skin quality
- Examples: Red peppers, raspberries, watermelon, grapes, and beets

Orange and Yellow Produce

- Main benefits: Improves immune function, reduces heart disease risk, and promotes eye health
- Examples: Oranges, sweet potatoes, and orange and yellow peppers

Green Produce

- Main benefits: Boosts your immune system, helps detoxify your body and restores energy and vitality
- Examples: Broccoli, Swiss chard, arugula, kale, and spinach

Blue and Purple Produce

- Main benefits: Fights cancer and inflammation
- Examples: Blueberries, purple cabbage, eggplant, prunes, and figs

White and Brown Produce

- Main benefits: Protects against certain cancers, keeps bones strong, helps your heart
- Examples: Cauliflower, garlic, potatoes, and jicama

TAKE A YEARLY VACAY

Go pack that suitcase. Not only can vacations improve heart health, they can also add years to your life. Here's the surprise, though: you don't need a vacation to feel happy. Just planning or anticipating an upcoming trip can make you happier than actually taking it.

Vacationing every year reduced the risk of death from heart disease by as much as 30 percent, according to a study from the State University of New York at Oswego. Meanwhile, women who vacationed at least twice a year were less likely to die of a heart attack than women who just got away once every six years. Those non-vacationing women were actually eight times more likely to have a heart attack than women who vacationed.

While those might be the most compelling reasons to vacation, they're not the only ones. Vacations can promote health by helping you start good habits like sleeping or moving more. And if you're struggling to get your weight down, research has linked vacations to lower waist circumference and body mass index. They can even decrease depression and make you happier.

GREEN YOUR GRILLING

Time to quit grilling meat and turn to veggies instead. Cooking meat at high temperatures creates substances called polycyclic aromatic hydrocarbons (PAHs) and heterocyclic amines (HCAs). Lab experiments show that PAHs and HCAs can cause changes in your DNA that could increase cancer risk. But you don't get PAHs just from eating the meat. When you're standing around a barbecue, your skin also picks up the PAHs, and although clothes can protect you, once they become saturated with barbecue smoke, your skin can take in high amounts of PAHs.

The best way to avoid this? Grill green, like the American Institute for Cancer Research suggests. Grilling fruits and veggies produces no dangerous compounds, and numerous studies have found that diets high in plants can help lower your cancer risk.

If you can't live without grilled meat, however, at least reduce cooking time over the flames by partially cooking any meat in a microwave, oven, or stove before placing it on a preheated grill. Trimming the fat and marinating meat in pilsner beer (even if it's non-alcoholic) lower the levels of PAHs. Also, if you've been around a grill, wash your clothes soon after leaving to reduce your exposure to PAHs.

CRAFT A LIFE PURPOSE STATEMENT TO IMPROVE WELL-BEING

Having purpose doesn't only give you more motivation to get out of bed every morning, it could also help you live longer. One of the most telling pieces of evidence to support this comes from a study of 9,050 people, averaging sixty-five years old. Those with the greatest well-being (as measured by questions that asked about the sense of control, life purpose, and feeling that what you're doing is worthwhile) were 30 percent less likely to die over the eight-and-a-half-year follow-up period than their peers with the lowest well-being. They also lived an average of two years longer than those with the lowest well-being.

So how do you find your purpose in life? Ask yourself what you love to do most, when you've experienced the greatest joy, and what you are most passionate about in life. Now draft a statement about how you want to live your life, based on that passion, and follow it daily.

FAST FOR TWELVE TO FOURTEEN HOURS A DAY

You fast every night when you go to bed, so why not extend that fast a little longer? This "intermittent fasting" could add years to your life and improve your health. Intermittent fasting is an umbrella term for any type of fasting that cycles between eating and not eating during a defined period, be it long or short. There's still a lot that researchers need to unearth about intermittent fasting, but so far, studies are showing that it may decrease risk factors related to aging, diabetes, cardiovascular disease, and cancer.

One of the easiest ways to try intermittent fasting is to do what's called "early time-restricted feeding," where you fast for twelve to fourteen hours between dinner and breakfast. Not only does that encourage you to eat earlier in the day, which gives you a metabolic boost, you're also fasting when you're sleeping, so you're less likely to experience hunger pangs. Finish your last meal about two hours before you go to bed to give your body time to digest the food; then wait for twelve to fourteen hours to eat again.

DON'T SIT FOR MORE THAN THIRTY MINUTES AT A TIME

Bet you've heard that sitting is the new smoking. And it's true—to some extent. Sitting too long really can kill you, even if you're a devout gym-goer. When you sit for prolonged periods—research indicates that people spend 50 to 60 percent of their waking hours, or about eight to ten hours a day, sitting down—your body begins to shut down metabolically. The rate at which your fat cells produce fat accelerates. Blood flows more slowly throughout your body when you sit, which makes it more likely that fatty acids will add to plaque build-up in your heart's vessels. Sitting even compromises blood flow in your lower extremities, which can create dangerous conditions like deep vein thrombosis. And because you're not burning as many calories as when you're moving or standing, you risk gaining weight.

Bottom line? Sitting for prolonged periods of time is a risk factor for early death, and that risk increases the more you sit. According to a study in *Annals of Internal Medicine*, for folks sitting more than thirteen hours a day, their risk of death was 200 percent greater than those sitting for less than eleven hours a day. Even folks who exercised regularly weren't off the hook.

Research suggests that limiting sit time to fewer than thirty minutes is the best practice. Set a timer every thirty minutes if you must, whether you're in the office or at home, and take a five-minute standing break. Bonus points if you incorporate movement (think simple stretches, walking, or climbing stairs) into that break.

EMBRACE MEATLESS MONDAYS

Cutting meat from your diet could be a big skin—and life—saver, even if you just do it once a week. Animal protein not only contributes to an early death, it also ages your skin. It might sound crazy to think that meat could lead to wrinkles, but remember that food can influence every organ in your body, including your skin. In the Food Habits in Later Life study of 2,000 people over seventy, those who frequently ate red meat, especially processed meat (think hot dogs, ham, bacon, sausage, and some deli meats), had more wrinkles than those who rarely consumed meat.

Animal protein damages other organs too. Eating too much red meat and not enough veggies could increase your body's biological age and contribute to health problems. Processed meat is also a carcinogen, meaning that it causes cancer, and red meat is a probable carcinogen. Saturated fat from animal products can even age your brain and cause an early death.

If cutting animal protein completely is too radical for you, adopt the Meatless Monday habit. The global movement, started in 2003 by the Johns Hopkins Bloomberg School of Public Health, encourages individuals to go meatless on Mondays. For more information, visit www.meatlessmonday.com.

GET BRONZED SANS THE SUN

Three words you need to hear: tanning beds kill. Unless you want premature skin aging and a higher risk of potentially fatal skin cancer, you'll run from tanning beds and switch to sunless tanners. Tanning beds might seem like a "healthy" alternative to outdoor tanning—after all, you're out of the sun, and you're building that base tan, right? Wrong. The radiation you get from those beds is similar—and in some cases, stronger—than that of the sun. Just ten minutes of being in a tanning bed is equivalent to ten minutes of being in the Mediterranean sun in summer, which may be why indoor tanners are 74 percent likelier to develop the deadliest form of skin cancer, melanoma, than folks who have never used one of these beds. Plus, people who visit tanning beds are 2.5 times more likely to have squamous cell carcinoma and 1.5 times more likely to have basal cell carcinoma. And if you use a tanning bed before turning thirty-five, your risk for melanoma increases by 75 percent.

Besides, the concept of a base tan is false. Any change in your skin color indicates skin damage, which can up your risk of potentially deadly skin cancer and causes premature aging.

Still want that bronzed look? Try a sunless tanner. The active ingredient, dihydroxyacetone, combines with amino acids in your skin to cause browning. Although there's some concern about inhaling it, it's safer than UV rays. While you can get a professional spray tan, you can also use a self-tanner at home. After exfoliating, apply the tanner to dry skin evenly in a thin layer and wait fifteen minutes until it dries. Wash your hands so your palms don't stain, and remember that you still need to use sunscreen.

KEEP YOUR HANDS LOOKING YOUNG

You might be able to hide your age in your face with makeup, but your hands are harder to cover up. They're more exposed to the sun than any other part of your body, which is why wrinkles and brown spots appear faster here than on other body parts. Solution? Sunscreen repeatedly applied frequently throughout the day.

Science confirms that hands are one of the easiest places to identify aging. A study in the journal *Plastic and Reconstructive Surgery* revealed that most people can accurately tell a person's age by looking at their hands. The youngest-looking hands were characterized by fullness and a lack of wrinkles and veins. While you'll have to talk with a surgeon about bothersome veins in your hands, you can at least apply sunscreen with SPF 30 to reduce the potential for sunspots. Reapply several times a day to counter what you lose when you wash your hands.

Other options to treat wrinkled hands include lotion containing retinol or glycolic acid (which you apply before bedtime), a light chemical peel every one to three months, and laser treatment, which can also help diminish age spots, according to the American Academy of Dermatology. Ask your dermatologist which of these options might be best for you.

EAT SMALLER FISH

Because of its heart-healthy omega-3 fatty acids, eating fish can help reduce the risk of heart failure, coronary heart disease, cardiac arrest, and ischemic stroke (the most common kind of stroke), according to the American Heart Association (AHA). In fact, studies have found that the Mediterranean diet, which not only emphasizes plant-based foods but also fish, benefits the heart. Now add in the fact that people in the Blue Zones (the five places in the world where people not only live the longest but are also the healthiest) eat fish up to three times a week. The AHA recommends eating two 3.5-ounce servings of non-fried fish or about ¾ cup of flaked fish every week for better health.

One caveat to remember is the environmental concerns about fish. Oceans are being overfished, and lots of modern-day fish are contaminated with pesticides and other chemicals (like mercury). If you do want to eat fish (and you're not pregnant), choose smaller, oily types, like salmon, anchovies, mackerel, herring, lake trout, and sardines. Watch out for sushi tuna, which studies show contains high amounts of mercury, and avoid farm-raised fish. Want to have your fish without actually eating it? Companies like Good Catch, Ocean Hugger Foods, and New Wave Foods have created "fish" made out of plants, including chickpeas, lentils, soy, sea algae, and tomatoes. Many of them are already available in grocery stores, so keep your eyes open.

ENJOY A ROLL IN THE HAY

Here's an anti-aging tip that's fun to implement: having sex could keep you looking younger. In a study of 3,500 individuals, those who had sex 50 percent more than average looked anywhere from four to seven years younger (average frequency for twenty- to thirty-year-olds was four times a week, while three times a week was average among individuals aged forty to fifty). One important note—most of these individuals had higher levels of physical activity than most people to begin with, and that factor was more important than the sexual factor.

Still, having sex frequently is certainly something to consider, as researchers found that good sex leads to pleasure and happiness in a relationship, thus fewer crow's-feet and frown lines. Sex also improves circulation and releases beneficial substances like oxytocin, beta-endorphins, human growth hormone, and in men, testosterone, which all have beneficial effects, especially in the long term. (As an aside, studies have also found that frequent ejaculation can help reduce a man's risk of prostate cancer.)

One important point, though? While the lovemaking is good, love is even better. If your sex life with your partner has taken a plunge, it's time to chat about it. Even putting sex on a to-do list could help reignite the flames.

EAT THE DAILY DOZEN

The book *How Not to Die* suggests that you should be eating eleven specific foods every day to prolong your life. This *New York Times* bestseller is by Dr. Michael Greger, a nutrition researcher and healthy-eating guru who runs www.nutritionfacts.org. It distills healthy eating—all for the sake of achieving not just a long but also a disease-free life—into easy-to-swallow morsels of information, namely the eleven healthiest foods you should eat every day, supplemented by exercise. The key ingredient? All of them are plants, which Dr. Greger believes add years to your life and life to your years.

Here's your Daily Dozen checklist:

1. Beans—3 servings
2. Grains—3 servings
3. Berries—1 serving
4. Other fruits—3 servings
5. Greens—2 servings
6. Vegetables—2 servings
7. Cruciferous vegetables—1 serving
8. Flaxseed—1 serving
9. Nuts—1 serving
10. Spices—1 serving
11. Beverages (water, green tea, hibiscus tea)—1,750 ml
12. Exercise—90 minutes moderate or 40 minutes vigorous

You can also download Dr. Greger's Daily Dozen app for free and track your daily servings on your phone.

RE-ESTABLISH GOOD SLEEP HABITS

Without proper sleep, your skin ages, your health crumbles, and you may not live as long—which is why you need to work on getting seven to nine hours every night. Here's sleep's surprising link to skin: sleeping for six hours just five nights in a row doubles the number of fine lines and wrinkles and increases brown spots and dark circles under the eyes. If too little sleep were to become your standard, all of those effects could worsen, triggering premature skin aging and permanent skin discoloration.

Studies have also shown that inadequate sleep contributes to heart disease, cancer, diabetes, and obesity; impairs learning and memory and raises your risk of Alzheimer's; weakens your immune system so you're more vulnerable to colds and the flu; affects your physical and mental performance; contributes to depression and other mental health disorders; and can even cause an early death. The list goes on, but suffice it to say that if you're among the one in every three Americans not getting the sleep you need, your health will suffer. Sleep, after all, is the only time your body has to heal—just ask any athlete about the powers of sleep— and without that time, negative consequences will result.

The National Sleep Foundation recommends that individuals older than eighteen log seven to nine hours of sleep a night. To help you achieve that, stick with a consistent bedtime and wake-up time, even on weekends; establish a relaxing bedtime ritual like taking a bath or meditating; avoid napping in the afternoons if you're having trouble sleeping; exercise daily; and sleep in a cool, dark, noise-free room.

GET OUT OF BED IF YOU CAN'T SLEEP

Trouble staying asleep? As odd as this sounds, get out of bed. You need to sleep if you want to age gracefully, and this is the best trick in the book if you're struggling with sleep. Waking in the middle of the night is one of the most common sleep problems, and it can get worse as you get older. One study found that older adults aged sixty and up are four times more likely to wake up throughout the night, versus young adults aged twenty-one to thirty years.

The solution might be counterintuitive, but it's one every sleep doc will sign on to: get out of bed and do something relaxing like read a real book (if you read from a tablet, the light from the screen could worsen your sleep woes) or listen to music. Don't turn on the TV or the blue light from the screen will suppress melatonin production, which signals your body that it's time to sleep. When you feel sleepy, head back to bed, trying not to look at the clock as you go. Continue repeating this as many times as you need during the night until you're finally back to sleep.

By removing yourself from the bed, you prevent your brain from thinking of bed as "bad," and you'll be able to slip back into slumber and wake up looking refreshed and raring to go, versus haggard and aged. One caveat? This strategy is best for people dealing with short-term sleep issues, not ones that have lasted longer than three months.

PUMP SOME IRON

Lifting weights isn't just for bodybuilders, Olympic athletes, or men. If you want to keep your muscles looking young and supple via tone and definition, you'll strength train two to three times a week. Loss of muscle mass and strength, something called sarcopenia, is a natural part of aging. You generally lose 5 to 7 pounds of muscle every decade of your adult years, which can decrease resting metabolic rate, or the rate at which your body burns calories, by 3 to 5 percent. This is one reason people typically gain weight and body fat as they age. Reduced muscle strength can also increase disability, interfere with your ability to walk and do other activities, and make you more vulnerable to falls. Yet all of this can be prevented through a regular strength training program.

Bonus? Strength training not only helps maintain and build bone density (which is key if you're at risk for osteoporosis), it also helps increase metabolism and decrease fat. That slimming effect will allow your muscles (for example, in common trouble spots like upper arms, thighs, and abs) to look more defined, giving you a more youthful appearance.

Aim to do strength training two to three times a week on non-consecutive days (your muscles need that time to rest), completing two to three sets of eight to twelve repetitions per exercise (if you're pressed for time, just do one set). And don't worry if you don't belong to a gym and can't access strength training machines. Other equipment may do a better job training your body, and you can stock all of it in a home gym. Consider dumbbells, resistance bands, stability balls, kettlebells, medicine balls, and TRX equipment.

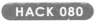

BOOST YOUR FIBER INTAKE WITH A SALAD APPETIZER

Here's an easy Rx for living longer (and looking and feeling good while doing it): eat more fiber by starting meals with a leafy green salad or brothy veggie-based soup. Fiber is the nondigestible carbohydrate in plants. If you're on the burger-and-fries diet, you're no doubt missing out, which explains why the average American only gets 14 grams of fiber a day. If, however, you're eating a plant-heavy diet, you'll have no trouble getting the fiber that you need.

Why is fiber so important? Research indicates that people who eat more fiber have fewer chronic diseases, as fiber can reduce your risk of heart disease, type 2 diabetes, and some cancers. And by adding more fiber to your diet, you can lose weight without making any other changes.

Dietary guidelines recommend that women eat at least 25 grams a day if they're under fifty, while women fifty-one and older need 21 grams. For men, recommendations are at least 38 grams if you're younger than fifty and at least 30 grams a day if you're fifty-one or older.

Choose fiber-rich foods over fiber supplements for the healthiest option. (Talk with your physician if you opt for supplements, as they could interfere with the absorption of some medications or may not be appropriate if you have certain medical conditions.) Also, make sure you go slowly when adding fiber to your diet. If your body isn't used to the high fiber intake, it can cause uncomfortable side effects like bloating, cramping, and gas at first. Once your body adapts, however, these issues usually disappear.

EAT YOUR BIGGEST MEAL FIRST

Got weight woes? Here's an easy solution that might help shave off some of that weight so it doesn't shave years off your life: make breakfast (or whatever your first meal is) your biggest.

This is obviously a huge change for most folks, who chomp their biggest meal in the evening. Here's why it's not a great idea: going to bed with a full tummy can disrupt sleep, and if you've eaten food that triggers heartburn, that can make sleep even more difficult. Besides, how often are you going for a walk or doing any type of movement after dinner? Chances are, you're probably retiring to the couch, making it unlikely that you'll burn off any of the calories you just ate.

Yet by flipping your meals around so that you're eating your heaviest meal first—in other words, you adhere to the adage of eating like a king at breakfast, a prince at lunch, and a pauper at dinner—you could drop pounds and a belt size (or two). In one study from the *Journal of the American College of Nutrition*, women who consumed 70 percent of their calories during breakfast, a morning snack, and lunch lost more weight and body fat than women who ate 55 percent of their calories during the same time frame.

Other benefits include improving blood sugar control and blood pressure, so why not try it? At the very least, finish eating your last meal of the day about two hours before bed so that you give your body time to digest.

SET UP A SLEEP SANCTUARY

Getting enough sleep is a great way to ensure overall health and well-being. To make sure you're sleeping soundly each night, create an environment that promotes sleep. Start by eliminating the TV and all digital devices from your room—your bed should be reserved for sleep and sex only. If you must sleep with a smartphone in your room, place it out of reach from your bed (so you're less tempted to check it during the night) and quit using these devices thirty to sixty minutes before bed. You should also dim the lights in your bedroom about an hour before you try to sleep.

Next, check that your room is dark—use blinds or blackout shades if necessary—and cool. Ideal sleeping temperature is between 60°F and 67°F, according to the National Sleep Foundation. The color of your room might even matter. A Travelodge survey found that people who slept in a blue room logged the best night's sleep. Other colors that induced better sleep included yellow, green, silver, and orange. Colors that were the least favorable to sleep? Purple, brown, and gray.

Reduce noise around your bedroom as much as possible, too, and be sure to never fall asleep with the TV on. Using a fan or white noise machine that provides a consistently soothing background all night can help. If your partner's snoring or your pet's movements are keeping you up, try to address those distractions too.

SEEK HELP FOR DEPRESSION

Rates of depression in America are alarming. About one in six adults will experience depression at some point in his or her life. Although anybody can be affected, women are twice as likely as men to experience depression, and aging can increase your risk of developing depression. It's such a serious health condition that the World Health Organization concluded that depression can be even more damaging to health than arthritis, asthma, diabetes, and angina.

While everybody has bouts of sadness every now and then, depression is more than just a bad day. There are more than fifty symptoms of major depression, but the main ones include feeling sad or anxious all the time; not wanting to do activities that used to be fun; eating more or less than normal or not having any appetite; being tired despite sleeping well; having trouble sleeping; feeling irritable or easily frustrated, even worthless or helpless; and thinking about committing suicide or hurting yourself.

If you (or somebody you know) are suffering from depression, don't ignore it. Instead, seek professional help. Numerous therapies are available to help overcome depression.

HIIT IT

Exercise is a cornerstone of graceful aging. If you're pressed for time, try high-intensity interval training (HIIT). HIIT simply means alternating between periods of very hard work and periods of rest. With this type of exercise, you'll improve cardiovascular fitness, lower your blood sugar, and can even reverse signs of aging at the cellular level, preventing the loss of mitochondrial activity which typically declines with age and is associated with greater fatigue and a reduction in your muscles' ability to burn any excess blood sugar. Yet the real magic lies in the fat loss. Studies show that HIIT may be even more effective than traditional cardio in helping you shed fat, both the kind that you can pinch (subcutaneous) and toxic abdominal fat that surrounds your organs (visceral).

Perhaps the best thing about HIIT is that you need only ten to twenty minutes to do it, making it the perfect workout if you're short on time. There are many ways you can structure a HIIT workout. If you're fairly fit, try sprinting for thirty seconds in whatever activity you're doing, recovering for four minutes, and repeating again four to six times. If you need a less intense session, climb a hill during that thirty-second burst and then recover. Or, play with whatever work-to-rest ratio works for you, whether that's thirty seconds of hard activity followed by one minute of easy, one minute hard followed by one minute easy, or one minute hard followed by two minutes easy. If you have any joint issues, using a stationary bike is often easier than running or walking when doing HIIT. Because of its intense nature, do HIIT no more than one or two times a week, and, of course, check with your healthcare provider before adding it to your program.

SET A DAILY STEP GOAL

Being sedentary for most of the day, even if you're exercising for a thirty-minute period, can raise your risk of numerous diseases as well as early death. Setting a step goal that fits your lifestyle might motivate you to move more throughout the day, decreasing some of that sedentary time. While you've probably heard that you should take 10,000 steps a day, roughly five miles, this number isn't based on any scientific evidence. It may even be too lofty a goal for some people, considering that the average American takes 4,774 steps per day (worldwide, the average daily step count is 4,961 steps).

Instead, set a daily step goal you can achieve. First, figure out how many steps you're currently taking by wearing a fitness tracker or pedometer (pedometers are cheaper and may track steps better than fitness trackers, but it's a personal preference) for seven days. Figure out the total number of steps for those days and divide by seven to determine your daily average step count. Then set a goal to increase that number by 5 to 10 percent over several weeks. If you find that you can easily achieve that and feel good about the movement you're doing, continue gradually increasing your steps.

And don't think you're off the hook if you hit the gym five days a week. More research is showing that while structured exercise (where you raise your heart rate) is good, that alone won't keep the body and brain young, and in fact, what you do—or don't do—between those workouts is just as important.

USE AGE-LESS COOKING TECHNIQUES

Clearly, what you eat can contribute to your skin health. But here's something you may not know: *how* you cook food can cause skin aging, and might even damage your body internally. Unless, that is, you take the high and dry heat out of your cooking repertoire.

High and dry heat increases advanced glycation end products (AGEs) in your body, and that's not good. There are two ways you get AGEs: your body produces some, but the rest come from the foods you're eating (beef and cheese are especially bad culprits). Certain cooking methods (like cooking in high, dry heat) can then cause more AGEs to form. The consequence? Studies have linked AGEs to skin aging and a whole host of other diseases, including heart disease, type 2 diabetes, Alzheimer's, cancer, cataracts, and kidney disease.

Limit AGEs in your diet by eating more fruits, vegetables, and whole grains. Then change your cooking techniques by avoiding high and dry cooking as much as possible. Some strategies:

- Cook foods on lower heat and longer
- Choose cooking methods that allow foods to stay moist as they cook (think steaming, stewing, or poaching versus grilling, roasting, broiling, or frying)
- Marinate meats before cooking them
- Microwave foods, which actually produces fewer AGEs than using dry-heat methods
- Cook at home more often so you avoid processed foods, which often contain high amounts of AGEs

SPICE UP YOUR FOOD

What does spicy food have to do with living longer? Research shows that people who eat spicy food regularly—mainly from fresh and dried chili peppers, which contain a health-promoting ingredient called capsaicin— are also less likely to die from heart and respiratory diseases, even cancer, than people who eat spicy foods only every now and then. If you can tolerate spicy foods and don't have digestive issues that would be affected by spices, it can't hurt to add some heat to your meals.

Here's a quick and easy spicy scramble with tofu (see hack #117 for why you should enjoy soy): drain 14 ounces of firm or extra-firm organic tofu; then crumble with your hands, mash with a potato masher, or dice into cubes, depending on the texture you prefer. Chop any veggies you like (mushrooms, onions, peppers, and spinach, for instance) and sauté them for about five minutes in 1 tablespoon of either olive oil or veggie broth in a skillet over medium heat. Push veggies to one side of the skillet and add tofu. Meanwhile, stir together 1 teaspoon of cumin, 1 teaspoon of chili powder, $\frac{1}{2}$ teaspoon of sea salt, $\frac{1}{2}$ teaspoon of turmeric, $\frac{1}{4}$ teaspoon of black pepper, and a splash or two of water until it forms a paste. Add the spice mix to the tofu and cook for 2 to 3 minutes; then stir everything together. Add a few shakes of nutritional yeast, perhaps some cherry tomatoes, and drizzle hot sauce to your liking. Serve over a bed of spinach.

SAY NO THANKS TO RECEIPTS

Chemicals like BPA and BPS have found their way into paper receipts, like the type you get at the grocery store. An unbelievable 93 percent of paper receipts are coated with either BPA or BPS. When you handle those receipts, those chemicals are absorbed into your skin in seconds, something that should concern retail workers who might handle thousands of these receipts in a week's time. While 81 percent of Americans were found to have detectable levels of BPS in their urine in 2014—thermal paper receipts account for 90 percent of that BPS—retail workers have been found to have 30 percent more BPA in their bodies on average than other adults. BPA has been shown to contribute to neurological, developmental, and reproductive issues. BPS may have similar negative consequences.

That's why Green America is encouraging everybody to skip the slip. If you do take a receipt, reduce your exposure to the chemicals by folding it so the printed side is facing in. Then wash your hands right away, especially if you touch thermal receipts frequently. Even better, be a proactive consumer and ask companies to offer digital receipts or use nontoxic receipt paper. It's not just for your health, but also for the environment. Paper receipts use over 12.4 million trees, 13 billion gallons of water, and generate 1.5 billion pounds of waste annually.

DRINK GREEN TEA FOR SUPPLE SKIN

There are many good reasons to drink teas, but perhaps the best reason in terms of anti-aging? You can boost skin elasticity with green tea. A study from Texas Woman's University in Houston showed that sipping green tea beverages every day for twelve weeks improved skin elasticity in women. Women drank eight cups a day in the study, but drinking that much even just two to four days over several months will work. A powerful antioxidant in green tea called epigallocatechin gallate (EGCG) may help prevent wrinkles too. Green tea may even lower your risk of skin cancer, as EGCG can protect against UV damage and decrease inflammation associated with aging.

Plus, green tea has been shown to boost brain health, help you lose weight, and lower glaucoma and heart disease risk. Aim for at least two cups a day and stick with unsweetened versions and freshly brewed if possible (it contains more catechins than bottled tea and none of the calories or sugar that bottled teas often contain). Not a green tea fan? Try black or oolong tea.

USE YOUR FACE LOTION ON YOUR ARMS

Age brings on some of the weirdest conditions, including little blood spots on your arms that look like red dots. Like all of the rest of the skin on your body, your arm skin thins as you age. It's made worse if you've had chronic sun exposure throughout the years, which can damage your skin's support system, namely collagen and elastin, or if you're taking certain medications like prescription blood thinners, aspirin, or non-steroidal anti-inflammatories. All of this makes your arms more vulnerable to bruising—often what appears as little blood spots that usually disappear over time.

The best solution is to apply the anti-aging products you're using on your face to your hands and arms. Products that contain ingredients like retinol and peptides can help build collagen in your skin, and thicker skin with more collagen will have a tougher time bruising.

C THE CHANGE

You may have heard that vitamin C helps you avoid or get over a cold. But did you know that topical vitamin C can improve your skin too?

You should get your share of vitamin C from your diet, especially foods like oranges, mangoes, papaya, and yellow bell peppers (which surprisingly contain more vitamin C than oranges). By eating your vitamin C, you'll decrease signs of aging, improve skin color and skin tightness, and decrease wrinkles.

Double those benefits by using vitamin C topically on your skin. Although vitamin C isn't a sunscreen per se, one of its benefits includes protecting your skin against UV-induced damage. Even better? Studies have shown that when used topically, vitamin C can decrease skin roughness, increase production of collagen, and offer protection against accelerated wrinkling. Choose a serum to get vitamin C in its most concentrated form. Then use it under your sunscreen every morning to give your skin even greater protection not only against pollutants but the sun too.

MAKE A HOMEMADE LAVENDER SKIN MISTER

Lavender isn't just an herb to help you sleep. It can also be an ally for aged, dehydrated skin. Studies suggest that lavender oil, rich in antioxidants, can promote the healing of wounds because it helps collagen synthesize. That's also why it can have positive effects on aging skin, providing hydration and increasing circulation to bring a youthful glow to the skin.

Try making a lavender oil mist that you can spritz on your face whenever it needs a pick-me-up. Add 20 drops of lavender essential oil to 2 ounces of distilled water in a small spray bottle. Close your eyes, then mist your face or other areas of your skin as often as you need. You can even keep it in the fridge and use it on sunburns to help them heal and cool.

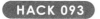

VOLUNTEER REGULARLY

Research shows that volunteering makes people not only happier but healthier. A European study found that volunteers are as healthy as non-volunteers five years younger. Talk about a positive way to turn back the clock! And indeed, studies have also found that people who volunteer may live longer than their non-volunteering counterparts with one caveat: your reason for volunteering should be about helping others instead of helping yourself.

You may not have much extra time in the week to spare on volunteering, and that's okay. Even just small amounts—as little as thirty minutes a week—are better than nothing, and plenty of organizations can use more hands on deck, no matter how much or how little time you have to give. Best part? You don't have to go anywhere physically if you're limited by time, resources, or geographic locations. You can lend that helping hand from the comfort of your home. To locate volunteer opportunities across the country, visit www.volunteermatch.org or contact an organization you're passionate about to learn how you can get involved.

HAVE FAITH

When it comes to living longer, faith matters. No matter what your spiritual or religious inclinations, having faith will help protect your brain from depression; this protection will boost your longevity. Yet having faith in general can also help you blow out more birthday candles.

For proof, turn to the Seventh-Day Adventists who live in Loma Linda, California, one of the five Blue Zones of the world. While these individuals follow lifestyle behaviors that would automatically add years to their lives (like not smoking, eating a plant-based diet, and having a strong sense of purpose), their faith may also be at play.

When Blue Zone centenarians were interviewed, all but five of the 263 surveyed were part of a faith-based community. More telling? Attending faith-based services about once a week (or four times a month) added four to fourteen years to their lives. Even those who attended service a minimum of one time a month reduced their risk of death by 30 percent. There wasn't a clear explanation of why having faith offers these benefits, but it could be related to a having a healthy support system.

CONSIDER FILLERS

Aging tends to come with a loss of fullness in the face, which can make you look tired and older. Loss of fullness, which starts as early as your thirties, shows up mainly in your cheekbones and chin. Blame the face-slimming, angular effect on a loss of collagen and hyaluronic acid, which your skin cells naturally make to help moisturize your face. When you hit your forties, you lose even more fat in your face, and because your skin isn't as resilient as it once was, it begins to look saggy.

That's why you might want to consider fillers. Fillers are considered a minimally invasive procedure that can plump your lips, diminish fine lines, and add fullness to cheeks and under your eyes by injecting your skin with ingredients that may include collagen, hyaluronic acid gel, and even fat from your own body. Fillers stimulate your body to make collagen, a protein that helps give your skin strength and elasticity, which can guard against future aging. Results from fillers are immediate and natural looking, and all it requires is a simple office visit. There are some side effects, but if you're working with a dermatologist or plastic surgeon—you don't ever want to do this in a non-medical setting—the negatives are minimal and may include redness, tenderness, swelling, and occasional bruising. Start with reversible fillers instead of permanent fillers. The reversible type uses hyaluronic acid, which can be easily dissolved if you don't like the results.

BE SKIN SAVVY WHEN INSERTING CONTACTS

Popping in contact lenses means that you're giving that skin around your eyes a tug several times a week, if not a day. Over time, that can wear the skin down. Because eye skin is so thin, it can easily damage, increasing the chance for wrinkles.

You still need to put in your contacts, of course. But being aware of your motions and seeing if you can limit how much you're moving that eye skin could really help. For instance, do you really need to extend your eyelid that far down or lift your eyebrows as high? Being more mindful of how you put your contacts in could help you use a more delicate touch. And hey, it's cool to wear glasses—so give that eye skin a break every now and then by sporting a pair of fashionable specs.

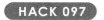

SLEEP ON YOUR BACK

Whenever you sleep on your side or stomach, you're creating unwanted lines in your face. Side sleepers usually end up with wrinkles on their cheeks and chin, while tummy dozers gain more wrinkles on their brow. Over time, those wrinkles can get deeper and become permanent.

Wrinkles aren't your only worry. Sleeping on your side can also make you lose facial volume or change the shape of your face on the side you sleep on. The effect is so pronounced that skin experts often say they can tell how you sleep just by looking at your face.

So sleep on your back if at all possible. If this causes your back to ache, slip a small pillow under your knees. If you can't stay in that position all night, use a pillow with a hole in the middle. It'll keep your head aligned and prevent you from rolling to your side.

If all else fails, at least switch sides every night—so if you sleep on your right side one night, sleep on your left the next to help balance out the loss of facial volume. Or when you're on your stomach, rotate your head from one side to another so you take pressure off your face.

BEWARE RUNNER'S FACE

Runners, you won't like hearing this news: although running can do wonders for your waistline, it's not so good for your skin. Everyone's skin will sag as they age, but those who run often see a negative impact on skin elasticity. Contrary to what you might think, though, it's not because you're pounding the pavement and gravity is causing that skin to sink. Instead, it's believed that oxidative damage from high-intensity sports, caused by less oxygen flow to your face, not only damages skin cells but also breaks down the skin's supporting fibers (collagen and elastin).

Plus, runners, especially those who are logging long distances, also sustain more sun exposure, which is why some studies have linked certain sports like running to increased skin cancer risk. That, plus weight loss, may explain why runners often have a more wrinkled appearance.

You don't have to give up your running routine, but do make sure you're wearing sunscreen whenever you run outside and try to run before 10:00 a.m. or after 4:00 p.m., as those are the times the sun is the most intense. You can also dial down your intensity while running, as studies have shown that the detrimental skin effects don't kick in until you're exercising at 70 to 80 percent of maximum heart rate. Even better? Swap a day of running with a lower-intensity exercise like walking, swimming, Pilates, or yoga—your muscles will also appreciate the chance to grow in new ways.

WALK FASTER

While any type of walking is good exercise, it turns out that walking faster is better for your health. Research suggests that walking speeds of faster than 1.0 meter/second (m/s) equate to healthier aging, while slower than .6 m/s increases the likelihood of poor health and function.

One reason? Walking places demands on numerous systems in your body, and a slowing gait could mean that one of those systems is damaged. It may also be an indication of de-conditioning, which can affect your health and longevity.

While many of these studies were conducted with older individuals, it doesn't hurt to work on your pace even when you're young. For starters, make sure you're doing aerobic activity, strength training, and flexibility work, all of which will give you the strength and endurance you need to walk. For pace specifically, focus on taking shorter steps and rolling from the heel to the ball of your foot, then push off again with your big toe.

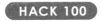

STAY IN HEALTHY BMI RANGE

Gaining weight doesn't only raise your risk of numerous health issues—it could also add years to your looks. In a study of 186 pairs of identical twins in the journal *Plastic and Reconstructive Surgery*, judges thought the overweight twin (who was about 24 pounds heavier than her sister) looked up to three years older. Researchers explain that while there was volume loss in some parts of the face with aging, with higher weights there was also an increase of fat deposits under the chin and development of jowls, which signal aging.

No matter your age, keep your weight around your ideal body mass index (BMI), because being overweight or obese increases the risk for thirteen different types of cancers. Keeping that weight stable isn't easy, but it's well worth your efforts. If you do try to lose weight, do so slowly. Otherwise, you may not get the nutrition and hydration that your skin needs, which could create a sunken appearance and make you look gaunt, frail, and, thus, older. Yet when you do lose, know this: for every 2.2 pounds of excess weight you lose, you'll increase lifespan by two months.

BOOST YOUR FRUIT AND VEGETABLE INTAKE

You really are what you eat, and by eating more fruit and veggies, you can fight wrinkles and get glowing skin. It's recommended that Americans eat 1.5 to 2 cups of fruits and 2 to 3 cups of veggies every day, but only 12 percent are eating enough fruit while only 9.3 percent are eating enough veggies.

Fruits and veggies don't just feed your body. They also nourish your skin, as they're filled with powerful antioxidants that protect your skin from sun damage, age spots, and wrinkles. They'll also aid skin growth and give your skin a healthy glow. Besides skin health, not getting enough fruits and veggies has other impacts on aging. Studies show that people who eat fewer than five servings of fruits and veggies a day had shorter telomeres than their produce-loving peers. The reason? Antioxidants in fruits and veggies stomp out free radicals, molecules that can damage cells and encourage telomeres to shrink more rapidly.

Aim to eat a minimum of five servings a day, although know that more is better. Eating raw, whole fruits and veggies is one easy way to increase your intake. Or try these strategies:

- Top your pizza with veggies
- Make a smoothie with fruits and veggies
- Swap zucchini noodles for pasta noodles
- Top your morning cereal with berries
- Make a PB&F (peanut butter and smashed fruit)
- Add frozen chopped spinach or kale to soups, stews, and sauces
- Use riced cauliflower in place of regular rice

GIVE THE SKIN AROUND YOUR EYES TLC

The skin around your eyes is so thin that it's ultra-prone to developing wrinkles, which is why you need to use a gentle touch whenever using skincare products on your eyes. The skin around your eyes actually ages faster than any skin on your face—hello, crow's-feet—and while sunscreen and sunglasses will help, this area also requires specific TLC.

Because that eye skin is so thin, it's more susceptible to UV damage and can easily be harmed with too rough a touch when applying skincare products and makeup. When you're using eye cream—you are using eye cream, right?—dab the eye product over the entire eye area, including under your eyes, above and below the brow bone, and in the corners of your eyes. Then use your ring finger to rub in the products, moving from your outside eye corners to your nose. Choose products that are specifically formulated for the eyes and include antioxidants as well as retinol.

ADD CONTRAST TO YOUR FACE

If you whip out your lipstick the second you finish eating a meal, you're helping yourself look younger. As you age, you lose facial contrast, meaning the contrast between your facial features and the surrounding skin, which makes you look older. Aging makes the lips, eyes, and eyebrows paler and the surrounding skin darker. Yet when cosmetics were applied to Caucasian women aged twenty to sixty-nine, facial contrast increased, which made them look younger, according to a study in *PLOS One*. Higher facial contrast also made faces appear healthier and more attractive than faces with lower contrast. Other studies have replicated this using women of different cultural backgrounds. In one study, greater facial contrast made Chinese, Latin American, South African, and French Caucasian women look younger 80 percent of the time.

So how can you increase facial contrast? Use mascara and eyeliner and darken your eyebrows. Applying lipstick, especially red, also does the trick.

MEDITATE FOR ONE MINUTE A DAY

If you want to dump stress (which is no doubt showing up on your skin), and even gain protection from aging on the cellular level, give meditation a shot for a single minute a day.

Studies show that regular meditation helps improve brain health, but it's also protecting you against aging on the cellular level. People with a longtime meditation practice—ten years in one study—have longer telomeres (the caps on your DNA strands) than people who have never meditated, and longer telomeres are associated with longer life.

You don't need to spend hours meditating every day to get the benefits. Even just *one* minute a day can give you the benefits of meditation. Once you find that you can set aside a minute a day—consider doing it before you get out of bed or right before you fall asleep—add a few more minutes until you're consistently doing between five and ten minutes a day. Just don't beat yourself up when your mind wanders, because it will. The main goal of meditation isn't to have your mind be entirely still. It's to train you to pull your mind back to the present every time it wanders away. As you get better at meditating, focusing becomes easier.

Whether you do guided or unguided is also a personal preference. It might be best to start with guided meditation, especially if you've never done it, and then move into unguided once you get comfortable with it. Try using apps like Calm and Headspace for assistance.

EAT MORE BLUEBERRIES

Good things really do come in small packages, namely blueberries. You wouldn't think a tiny fruit could pack such a nutritional anti-aging punch, but it can, which is why you should put a cup a day on your menu. Blueberries have been found to have the highest amount of antioxidants among all fruits and vegetables. Those valuable compounds fight disease-promoting free radicals in your body and skin.

Blueberries first earned superhero status for their effect on the memory. In fact, many brain experts list them among their top brain health foods because of their ability to decrease cognitive decline. Blueberries also lower blood pressure and may even have anti-cancer properties.

Plus, one serving (1 cup) of blueberries gives you almost 25 percent of your daily vitamin C requirements. As you'll remember from hack #91, vitamin C can increase collagen formation, giving you younger-looking skin. Not a blueberry fan? Raspberries and blackberries not only deliver similar benefits but also more vitamin C than blueberries. One cup of raspberries contains 54 percent of your vitamin C needs, while 1 cup of blackberries contains 50 percent.

CHERISH AT LEAST FIVE FRIENDS

It turns out that your friends aren't just good for your well-being because they're fun—they're also helping you live longer! When you think about all of the things friends do for you, it makes sense. They're the ones who lend a compassionate ear when life turns sour. They help lessen your stress. Friends make you happier, giving you that endorphin rush that can protect you from disease, and they care about your well-being, perhaps even leading you to healthier changes in life or supporting changes you're trying to make. On the flip side, people who are lonely have greater rates of depression and have a greater likelihood of dying from heart disease.

But how many friends do you need to achieve optimal well-being? A British researcher has deduced that the average person has roughly 150 social connections at any given point, but out of that group, only fifteen of the people closest to you are the most important for your overall well-being. Science has distilled it down even further to suggest that five is the perfect number of friends whom you should hold close.

REPLACE MEAT WITH MUSHROOMS

Mushrooms contain high quantities of two antioxidants that could unlock anti-aging powers in your body. All plants contain antioxidants, which fight oxidative stress in your body. That stress is caused by compounds called free radicals, which are produced by all sorts of things, including food, exercise, and stress. Your body can usually fight off these free radicals, but when they start accumulating, they can cause damage. They've been associated with heart disease, Alzheimer's, and cancer, to name a few.

Now back to those mushrooms. Research has found that mushrooms contain two antioxidants, ergothioneine and glutathione. People in other countries like France and Italy who eat more ergothioneine have lower rates of neurodegenerative diseases compared to people in the United States, who have a higher risk for diseases like Alzheimer's. One possible reason? Americans don't eat as much ergothioneine.

Plus, mushrooms can make you feel fuller longer (even more so than beef in some studies) and may even help you lose weight.

One of the easiest ways to get more mushrooms? Replace half (or more!) of the beef in homemade burgers with chopped mushrooms. Chances are, you won't even notice the difference. You can also use mushrooms instead of beef in spaghetti sauces and casseroles. Cooking mushrooms, by the way, doesn't change the levels of ergothioneine and glutathione, so don't worry about that.

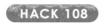

ENJOY THE MORNING LIGHT

While you don't *have* to rise in time to see the sun come up (although kudos if you do), getting a fifteen- to twenty-minute dose of morning light could do your body good. Not only could it help your body wake up—even better than a cup of coffee—studies have also linked getting natural light in the morning to sleeping better at night and helping you maintain a lower body mass index.

When it comes to sleeping, that morning light resets your circadian rhythms, helping your body and brain know when they should be awake and when they should be asleep. Research has proven that people who are exposed to higher amounts of light between 8:00 a.m. and noon typically sleep better: they fall asleep faster and stay asleep better than folks who see only low amounts of morning light.

Similar concepts apply to your weight. Syncing your body clock helps regulate your metabolism, which could be why morning light is a powerful ally in that battle of the bulge.

If possible, get outside every day between 8:00 a.m. and noon. Consider logging an outdoor workout during this time or just enjoying your cup of coffee outside for fifteen to twenty minutes. And don't let clouds scare you off. You're still getting light even if the day isn't meteorologically perfect.

GO NUTS

Blue Zone centenarians eat on average about two ounces, or two handfuls, of nuts a day. When it comes to the benefits of noshing nuts, heart health is perhaps the best known. Research shows that people who eat greater amounts of nuts have a lower risk of developing heart disease than folks who either never eat nuts or eat them infrequently. Even more telling? Another study revealed that eating animal protein was associated with a higher risk of heart disease—60 percent, to be exact—while noshing nuts (and seeds) for protein actually benefited the heart, lowering heart disease risk by 40 percent. Little wonder then that studies show that folks eating nuts outlive nut naysayers by two to three years on average.

Nuts are loaded with so many nutrients, including omega-3 fatty acids, magnesium, and copper, that their benefits even extend into lowering risk of death from cancer and respiratory disease. They've also earned some accolades for giving the brain a boost. Here's the biggest surprise: in spite of their high calorie content, nut eaters have consistently been shown to weigh less than non-nut eaters.

In case you need yet another reason to eat nuts, here's one: many nuts contain nutrients like vitamin E, selenium, and omega-3 fatty acids that could improve your skin. Unless you're allergic to them, there's no denying that nuts can aid your health—just enjoy them in moderation.

DIP INTO SOME HUMMUS

Hummus for a healthier America? That may be a fitting campaign slogan, given that hummus could extend your life and should factor into your weekly, if not daily, menu.

First, a hummus 101 lesson: Merriam-Webster defines hummus as "a paste of pureed chickpeas usually mixed with sesame oil or sesame paste and eaten as a dip or sandwich spread." Numerous food producers today are also making spreads from other beans, like white beans, edamame, and black beans, and calling them hummus (and yes, that has started a war of words, if you will).

Most Americans aren't eating enough vegetables, let alone legumes (you should be eating at least 1.5 cups a week). That's where hummus can come into play. Whether you use it as a dip for cut-up veggies or a spread for your wrap, hummus eaters naturally tend to have a higher-quality diet, eating more fiber than others and even more nutrients, like vitamins A, E, and C; magnesium; and potassium. Hummus might even help you manage your weight, improve markers of heart disease, aid with insulin regulation, and prevent certain cancers.

Ready to take a dip? Here are some other ways you can use hummus: use it in place of butter on a baked potato or mayo on a burger, make hummus soup, or add hummus in place of mayo in a chickpea salad.

TRY DIY SOLUTIONS FOR AGE SPOTS

Age spots are discolorations on your skin where the sun's rays have hit. Although they can pop up anywhere on your body, you'll most frequently find them on your hands and face.

The good news? Numerous treatment options for sunspots exist, namely creams and lotions or procedures like laser therapy and chemical peels. While you need to be diligent about using these creams and lotions—the American Academy of Dermatology (AAD) recommends using them once or twice a day for weeks to months—procedures like laser treatment, cryotherapy, microdermabrasion, or chemical peeling work faster.

An easier solution might be to use natural ingredients you already have in your kitchen—apple cider vinegar or pineapple—both of which have been reported to lighten skin. Mix equal parts apple cider vinegar with water and apply to the age spots, allowing the vinegar to sit for a few minutes before rinsing. Or, place a piece of pineapple on spots for fifteen minutes at a time, repeating each process at least once a day.

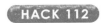

MAINTAIN TOP DENTAL HEALTH

You know that your teeth need regular check-ups to avoid cavities and gum disease (which is a surprising indicator of heart issues). But did you know that visits to the dentist can make you look younger too? As you age, your teeth start to wear down, making them shrink slightly in size. Larger teeth actually help support your lips, keeping them youthful. As time wears away at your teeth, lips lose their support and start sinking in, creating an aged appearance.

Work with your dentist to tailor a schedule based on your oral health. For people who are at low risk of periodontal disease, that might mean only one check-up per year. However, those at higher risk may need more frequent exams, as dentists can spot signs of tooth wearing and help you take action to prevent it, especially if you clench or grind your teeth, which can wear them down even more.

IMPROVE YOUR BALANCE

Falling is one potentially dangerous part of aging. A whopping one out of four individuals over sixty-five takes a fall at one time or another. Although falls can lead to broken bones and head injuries, most folks don't injure themselves too seriously when they fall, but they do become afraid of falling again. As a result, they limit their activities, which can wind up making them weaker.

Yet here's what you should know about falls: they're preventable, and the earlier you start working on your balance, even if you're only in your thirties, the greater the chance that you'll maintain that balance as you age.

To strengthen your sense of balance, do exercises that build muscle in your lower legs, and challenge your balance regularly by doing activities such as yoga, tai chi, or movements that throw your body off balance. Here's an easy one you can do anywhere, even while you're brushing your teeth or standing in line at the grocery store: stand on one leg for thirty seconds; then switch sides. To make this more challenging, do it with your eyes closed and/or move to a slightly unstable surface like a pillow or cushion.

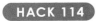

MOISTURIZE WITH SHEA BUTTER

Shea butter has often been called your skin's "best friend," namely because it has such exemplary moisturizing properties. It comes from the seed of a shea tree, hence its name, and one of its main components is vitamin A, which can help various skin conditions, wrinkles and dry skin included. Surprisingly, the moisturizers found in shea butter are the same ones that the sebaceous glands in your skin make, according to the American Shea Butter Institute.

In one study, the moisturizing effect lasted up to eight hours after its original application. Because of its antioxidants, shea butter has also been called an anti-inflammatory, and might be able to protect your skin from environmental irritants. Some studies even suggest that shea butter can increase collagen and decrease the appearance of wrinkles caused by sun exposure.

Look for shea butter that's raw and unrefined—in other words, a grade A shea butter. It comes in five grades ranging from A to E, and the American Shea Butter Institute recommends choosing grade A for optimal results. You can even check for the Institute's seal on any product you buy. Then use it as frequently as you need.

SWITCH TO AVOCADO BUTTER

Both butter and margarine increase your risk of skin wrinkling (not to mention a whole slew of health issues). Instead, use nature's butter: avocados.

Studies have shown that when people eat more butter and margarine (in one study, meat and dairy, too), they experience more skin wrinkling. Some of these spreads contain partially hydrogenated oils, which make the skin more prone to ultraviolet radiation, thus damaging your skin's collagen and elastin. They also cause chronic inflammation in the body, which can accelerate the formation of wrinkles.

Fortunately, nature has the perfect alternative that's packed with healthy fats, minerals, and vitamins: avocado. You can spread it on your toast as you would with butter or margarine, or when cooking use 1 cup of pureed avocado to replace 1 cup of butter. If you're baking, lower the oven temperature by 25 percent and increase the baking time.

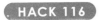

AVOID CANNED FOODS

Like most Americans, you probably have some canned food in your pantry. But here's a good reason to reconsider them: some cans contain the dangerous chemical BPA (bisphenol A), which is why you should limit or better yet, eliminate canned foods from your grocery list. BPA is considered a hormone disruptor and has been associated with numerous health conditions including heart disease, obesity, diabetes, and reproductive issues.

In one study that tested nearly 200 food cans on grocery store shelves, two out of three tested positive for BPA. Those who ate just one canned food in the past day had roughly 24 percent higher concentrations of BPA in their urine versus those who hadn't eaten canned food. That concentration of BPA increased by 54 percent with just two or more foods from cans. Another study found that eating canned soup and pasta resulted in higher BPA concentrations in urine than other foods, 229 percent for soup and 70 percent for pasta. Canned fruits and veggies, on the other hand, had 41 percent higher concentrations of BPA.

Researchers are still trying to determine the health consequences of BPA—and perhaps other chemicals that are replacing BPA, so don't assume "BPA-free" means "healthy"—but it's safe to say that the less canned food you eat, the better. Instead, opt for foods packaged in glass containers or fresh, unpackaged food as much as possible.

ADD SOY TO YOUR DIET

Soy is in the news frequently—it seems to be one of those foods that is good for you one day and bad the next. The research indicates this bottom line: soy is a health-promoting food that could help you live longer.

Soy contains phytoestrogens, plant-based compounds that share some of the same qualities as the hormone called estrogen. Because higher amounts of estrogen in the body have been associated with cancer, it is often assumed that soy is problematic—until you look at the research and realize that, as the Susan G. Komen organization states, "If there's one solid conclusion from all the data on soy and breast cancer, it's that eating moderate amounts of soy foods very likely does not increase the risk of breast cancer." Some studies even suggest that soy may help protect against breast cancer.

Consider this: in Asian countries where people tend to eat the highest amount of soy-based foods, breast cancer rates are lower than those in the United States. In Japan, people eat 25 to 50 milligrams (mg) of soy per day versus less than 3 mg in the United States, and researchers often point to soy as being one of the reasons breast cancer rates are lower in Japan.

Soy has also been shown to improve bone and heart health, help with weight loss, and perhaps protect against prostate cancer. Looking for protein sources outside of animals? Soy's got you covered: it's the only plant protein equivalent to animal protein, as it contains all nine essential amino acids.

Most of the research has been done on unprocessed or minimally processed soy foods like miso, edamame, tempeh, tofu, and soy milk, so choose those foods over more processed forms, including those that contain soy protein isolates. (Soy protein isolates originate from soybeans, but they are ultraprocessed and strip out other nutrients—plus, they're often genetically modified.) Soy supplements also won't get you the nutritional bang you're looking for, which is why it's best to stick with less processed soy foods.

HANG WITH HEALTHY FOLKS

Just like a cold, weight and even eating habits are contagious. So if you're trying to make a change on the scale, start hanging with your healthy-minded friends more.

This might sound like weird science, but it's a fact: obesity is contagious. There's something called social contagion, and studies have found that when more of the people you surround yourself with are obese, you then have a greater chance of being obese. Take, for instance, one study that looked at military families. When these families moved to counties with high obesity rates, they were then more likely to be obese or overweight. The opposite was also true. Even more telling? One study revealed that if one of your friends becomes obese, your likelihood of becoming obese increases by 47 percent (compare that to only 40 percent or 37 percent if your sibling or spouse, respectively, becomes obese). One explanation? You often model your own behaviors on your friend's actions. Plus, having an obese friend may make being overweight more acceptable.

Of course, this doesn't mean you should ditch your friends based on their weight alone, but if you're hoping to slim down and adopt healthier habits like eating better or exercising more, find more healthy folks to hang around so their habits rub off on you.

QUIT SQUINTING

You can't walk around stone-faced, but if you're constantly squinting, you'll make yourself look older. Facial motions like squinting make your muscles contract, causing the skin to wrinkle. Do this repetitively, and those wrinkles will become even deeper.

Various factors might cause you to squint, including being out in the sun and not being able to see the TV or your computer well enough. Whatever the reason, it's important to try to stop it from happening. Always wear sunglasses whenever you're outside, especially if you're in the sun. Get your eyes checked regularly, as squinting may mean that your vision's not as sharp as it once was. Also, take frequent breaks from screens, which can be tough on the eyes.

MEET YOUR MAGNESIUM NEEDS

Most Americans aren't getting enough magnesium, yet it is such a vital nutrient that your cells can't function without it. Magnesium plays a role in the more than 300 enzymes in your body, which do everything from producing energy and contracting muscles to keeping your bones and heart healthy. Even more importantly in terms of anti-aging, magnesium is crucial for your skin. When levels of magnesium in your body get too low, your skin loses fatty acids, which can reduce moisture and elasticity. Magnesium even plays a role in collagen formation and reducing acne, so without enough on board, your skin will undoubtedly suffer.

Guidelines recommend 400 milligrams (mg) a day for men aged nineteen to thirty, and 420 mg for men thirty-one and over, while women aged nineteen to thirty should get 310 mg a day and 320 mg if they're thirty-one or older. However, data indicates that men are only getting about 350 mg a day and women about 260 mg a day. If you're among that group, you could be missing out on valuable health benefits.

One study revealed that folks eating the highest amount of magnesium had a 10 percent lower heart disease risk, 12 percent lower stroke risk, and 26 percent lower risk of type 2 diabetes, versus folks eating the least amount. Just eating an extra 100 mg per day could even reduce diabetes risk by 19 percent and stroke by 7 percent. Magnesium has also been shown to improve sleep. Plus, by eating enough magnesium, you will help your body maintain its collagen production, preventing wrinkles and skin sagging.

Get your magnesium intake through food versus supplements. Good sources include dry-roasted almonds (80 mg in one ounce), boiled spinach (78 mg in ½ cup), plain soy milk (61 mg in 1 cup), cooked black beans (60 mg in ½ cup), and smooth peanut butter (49 mg in 2 tablespoons).

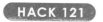

MAKE YOUR OWN NATURAL CLEANERS

Studies by the Environmental Protection Agency (EPA) have found that homes have two to five times the amount of roughly a dozen common volatile organic compounds (VOCs) than is found outside. One of the common sources? Cleaning products.

There's good reason to stay far away from VOCs. In the short term, you might experience symptoms like headaches, fatigue, dizziness, conjunctival irritation, nose and throat discomfort, and nausea. None of that sounds fun, of course, but even worse are the more serious issues like damage to the liver, kidneys, and central nervous system. Some of these toxins are "suspected or known to cause cancer in humans," the EPA states. Many of them can cause cancer in animals too.

So what should you use to clean? Items that you may already have at home! Green America lists ten common products that you can use to clean almost anything: white vinegar, baking soda, borax, hydrogen peroxide, club soda, lemon juice, liquid castile soap, cornmeal, olive oil, and pure essential oils. Here's an easy recipe for a multipurpose cleaner, which has a soothing scent to boot: mix 1 cup water with 1 cup white or apple cider vinegar and 10 to 20 drops lavender essential oil.

DON'T GET BAGGED DOWN

Too many of us lug around various bags that weigh us down. Whether it's a gym bag, shoulder bag, or messenger bag, carrying around too much weight can shift your posture and make you look older. The average woman's purse weighs 5 pounds, the equivalent of a bag of Domino sugar. Besides being awfully uncomfortable, numerous reasons should prompt you to avoid carrying heavy bags. Those bags can cause pain in your shoulders, neck, elbows, and back, and lead to more serious issues like changes in your walking gait. Heavy purses and bags can even change your posture, causing you to jut your head forward and round your shoulders. Upshot? You look older.

You don't have to give up that purse or shoulder bag entirely, but you should get smarter about how you pack it and carry it. The American Occupational Therapy Association recommends choosing purses with built-in compartments so you can distribute weight more evenly; making sure the bag is in proportion to your body size and comes with wide, adjustable straps; and avoiding bags made of heavy material like leather. When packing your bag take out duplicate items, kick coins out of your wallet, find travel-sized options for things like hand sanitizers, take only the keys you need, and pack fewer accessories. Also, switch to a backpack, when possible, or at least change shoulders frequently if you have to use a shoulder-slung bag.

SOOTHE DRY EYES

Your skin isn't the only organ that gets drier as you age. Your eyes also dry out as well. Although dry eyes are most common in people over sixty, they can start at any age. Things that can increase your risk include being a woman; side effects from medications (especially antihistamines, blood pressure medications, antidepressants, and decongestants); medical conditions like rheumatoid arthritis and diabetes; exposure to dry climates, wind, and smoke; contact lenses; and looking at screens too long without blinking. Dry eyes can cause your vision to be affected, and if you're a contact lens wearer, you might have more trouble wearing lenses.

For long-term relief, you can ask your optometrist about prescription medications or try over-the-counter drops. Taking an omega-3 supplement and looking away from screens every few minutes can also help.

More immediately, apply a warm compress to your eyes to stimulate oil glands in your lids. You'll moisturize your eyes and decrease symptoms of dry eye, making your eyes less itchy and less prone to being rubbed. You can either buy microwavable, reusable eye compresses or make your own. Just heat a bowl of water in the microwave until it's warm (but not hot or you'll scald your eyelids). Dip a washcloth in it and, with your eyes closed, gently massage the washcloth over your eyes for ten minutes. Repeat daily.

REAPPLY SUNSCREEN EVERY TWO HOURS

Putting sunscreen on in the morning is great, but you're not done for the day. You need to reapply this powerful defense against aging every two hours. This advice might sound like it's best reserved for those beach vacations or lazy days around a pool. While it applies there, too, it's also something you should start doing every day, whether you're going to the office or running your kids around.

Because sunscreen easily wears off and can be broken down by the sun, you need to reapply at least every two hours (although if you've just been swimming or sweating heavily, you'll need to reapply immediately). Set a timer on your phone to remind you throughout the day and then stash sunscreen sticks or bottles in your purse, office drawer, and glove box (unless it's too hot in your car, as the heat will cause sunscreen to break down more quickly) for reapplications.

MINIMIZE CROW'S-FEET WITH SOY MILK

While crow's-feet are a sign of a joyful life, you might not like how they look. Crow's-feet are those little fine lines that run from the corners of your eyes outward, and although they do indicate that you've smiled a lot, they can be one of the first—and most annoying—signs of aging.

While Botox is an effective treatment, so, too, is soy milk. You can certainly drink soy milk—studies are showing that one serving a day of soy milk has potential benefits for the skin, including decreasing wrinkles and the depth of wrinkles and helping with dryness, elasticity, coarseness, and pigmentation—or you can apply it on your skin. Doing so can increase your skin's elasticity, thicken thinning skin, and moisturize the skin to soften those crow's-feet. It can also help de-puff your eyes. Just soak two cotton balls with soy milk and, while lying down, place them over your eyes for roughly five minutes.

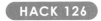

ADOPT A "LOW-RISK" LIFESTYLE

Americans rank a dismal thirty-first in life expectancy in the world. Yet adopting five habits could turn that around. These five habits were culled after researchers studied 123,000 Americans for over thirty years in an attempt to understand why Americans have one of the world's shortest lifespans compared to other high-income countries. While the behaviors themselves aren't new, it's the combination of all five that makes the magic.

Researchers call them "low-risk," and they include the following: not smoking, maintaining a low body mass index, doing at least thirty minutes of moderate to vigorous exercise every day, keeping alcohol intake to moderate levels, and eating a healthy diet. That diet was defined, by the way, as high in fruits, vegetables, whole grains, nuts, polyunsaturated fats, and omega-3 fats and low in sugary beverages, trans fat, sodium, and red and processed meats.

So just how many extra years could all of these five lifestyle hacks earn you? If you're fifty and adopt all five habits, you could live another 43.1 years if you're a woman and 37.6 years if you're a man. If you're not following these habits and you're fifty, give yourself only 29 more years of life if you're a woman, 25.5 years if you're a man.

TREAT ADULT ACNE NATURALLY

If you think acne is only a teenage issue, think again. Whether you're in your twenties, thirties, forties, or fifties, adult acne can strike anybody, even if you've never had it before. Women tend to experience adult acne at higher rates than men because of hormonal issues. But other contributing factors can include stress, hair and skincare products, family history, side effects from medications, and even a medical condition that's not yet diagnosed.

While you can see a dermatologist, you can also go natural and use tea tree oil, often used to treat wounds because of its antibacterial nature. Just mix about four to eight drops of tea tree oil with jojoba or coconut oil (don't apply tea tree oil directly, as it could irritate your skin). Dab the mixture on your problem areas.

SING!

If you start belting out tunes like there's no tomorrow whenever you get in your car or shower, you'll have many more tomorrows. That's because singing makes you smile, and when you smile, you're happier, and being happy can lead to a longer life. Singing was actually one of three activities Scandinavian researchers pinpointed as leading to a healthy, happy life (camping and dancing were the other two).

The benefits of singing are both physical and psychological. Surprisingly, singing counts as an aerobic activity, increasing oxygen in your blood and exercising all of the muscles in your upper body. Upshot? You could improve your breathing. On the mental side, it releases those feel-good hormones called endorphins that lift your mood and decrease stress, and because you're mentally exercising your brain, so to speak, you might even create new neural pathways, leading to less age-related cognitive decline.

Bottom line? Sing whenever the spirit moves you (let's hope it's often). Earn bonus points if you do it with others, as studies show this can give you a greater sense of well-being and community.

EMBRACE HUGGING

Not everybody in this world is a hugger. Hugging is even taboo in some cultures. Yet daily hugging—or holding hands or cuddling with a loved one—could help you live longer.

Physical contact with others, especially those whom you love, releases the hormone oxytocin, which can boost the immune system and help you fend off illnesses and even help you heal faster from wounds or reduce pain. Hugs will also de-stress you—one study found that people who were hugged had a huge decrease in the amount of the primary stress hormone, cortisol, in their bodies—and boost your self-esteem and happiness.

Because touch may be the first of our five senses to develop, it makes sense that touch plays such an integral role in health. How many hugs should you get a day? Take this advice from American psychologist and family therapist, Virginia Satir, to heart: "We need four hugs a day for survival. We need eight hugs a day for maintenance. We need twelve hugs a day for growth." Just make sure those hugs are firm or else that oxytocin may not be released.

LOOK SURPRISED

While you should still smile every day (it's good for happiness, after all), opt for a *surprised* look if you're trying to appear younger.

Even though the media is saturated with ads that portray smiling faces as being younger, researchers from Ben-Gurion University of the Negev were skeptical. So they asked individuals to rank photographs of people from oldest to youngest. Those photos included three different facial expressions: smiles, neutral expressions, and surprised looks. Guess which was ranked as the oldest? Smiles. On the flip side, the study participants agreed that surprised looks made people look youngest (neutral expressions ranked, unsurprisingly so, in the middle).

Here's the weird thing, though: study participants were asked to recall their reactions, and they incorrectly remembered smiling faces as being younger than faces with neutral expressions. Researchers say that smiling makes people look older because of crow's-feet, but when people look surprised, the skin gets pulled up and back, so any wrinkles are smoothed out. (Good thing to remember next time you're taking selfies to post to social media!)

FIGHT AGE SPOTS WITH TURMERIC

Turmeric, which turns curry yellow, contains compounds that people in India have regarded as medicinal for centuries. One of the main ones is curcumin, a strong antioxidant that has anti-inflammatory properties, helping your body fight diseases like cancer, rheumatoid arthritis, and heart disease. It can also improve the appearance of sun-damaged skin by lessening age spots and decreasing facial lines and wrinkles. In fact, using a cream with turmeric and niacinamide, a form of vitamin B3, was 15 percent more effective at reducing the appearance of fine lines and wrinkles versus a cream that used only niacinamide.

While you should add turmeric to your daily diet—eat ¼ teaspoon of turmeric a day in spice form or a quarter of an inch if you're eating fresh—you can also make your own solution at home to reduce age spots. Combine 1 teaspoon powdered turmeric with 2 tablespoons organic coconut oil and apply to your age spots several times a day until you get the results you want. Store the mixture in a sealed container for three to four days.

TONE FLABBY ARMS

Whether you call them bat wings or chicken wings, that jiggly flesh on the back of your arms can be a downer. Plus, extra flesh on your arms makes you look older. What gives? Simple: you lose muscle as you age. As that muscle tone disappears, your skin and fat are left with little internal support, so they hang. Gravity's also pulling the back of your arms, namely your triceps, down. That's where strength training comes into play. By building muscle in those triceps, you'll improve that muscle tone, helping your arms look firmer and more lifted as a result.

Try these three exercises to fight arm flab:

1. **Push-ups:** Get on your hands and knees, with your knees under your hips and your hands under your shoulders. If possible, lift your knees off the floor and hold your body in one long line as you do this. Keeping your abdominals contracted, lower your chest toward the floor as you keep your elbows as close to your sides as possible until you're about an inch or two off the floor. Push back up to start and repeat.

2. **Kickbacks:** Stand with your feet hip distance apart and a weight in each hand. Bending your knees slightly and leaning forward from your hips, lift your elbows behind you until your arms form 90 degree angles. Keep your elbows close to your body and press your hands behind you until your arms are extended. Release to start and repeat.

3. **Extensions:** Stand with your feet shoulder-width apart, holding one weight between your hands, with your arms by your thighs. Slowly lift the weight overhead. Keeping your shoulders down, abdominals engaged, and elbows close to your ears, bend your elbows and lower the weight behind your head. Release to start and repeat.

APPLY CABBAGE TO VARICOSE VEINS

Advancing age can make your veins become enlarged and look as if they're twisted and bulging. Those are the signs of varicose veins, which usually appear on the legs.

Yet age isn't the only factor, as issues with veins can start as early as your thirties. Obesity, pregnancy and hormonal changes, lack of movement, standing too much, genetics, and sun exposure can also increase your risk. While 50 to 55 percent of women have a vein issue, 40 to 45 percent of men do too.

Fortunately, you can take steps to prevent vein issues. Some tips: wear sunscreen, exercise regularly by doing leg-friendly activities like running and walking, control your weight, wear compression socks, avoid crossing your legs or sitting or standing for long periods of time, limit your time in high-heel shoes, and eat a high-fiber, low-salt diet.

But what if you already have visible varicose veins? Put some cabbage on them to help reduce pain and swelling. Chop cabbage leaves finely and add enough water to form a paste. Apply the paste to varicose veins and let it sit for several hours (wrap a linen cloth around your body part). Wash off the paste and repeat two times a day. Note, though, that you should always see your doc if you're having any issues with varicose veins.

RELIEVE ACHING MUSCLES WITH A FOAM ROLLER

You lose flexibility as you age, which makes moving tougher. While stretching is good, foam rolling is even better at keeping your muscles supple and young. A foam roller is a cylindrical-shaped tube that comes in various sizes. By lying on top of it and rolling it beneath you, you can massage your muscles, working deep into muscle tissue called fascia.

One of the main benefits of foam rolling is that you can reduce muscle soreness after exercising. Studies also show that foam rolling can increase the range of motion around the joints, reduce stiffness of the arteries, (even in healthy young adults), lower blood pressure, and reduce cellulite.

Foam rollers come in different firmness levels, so if you're new to foam rolling, start with one that's less firm. No matter what firmness you use, prepare to feel a little discomfort. It shouldn't be painful, though, so back off if it is. As you roll, notice areas that feel particularly tight. Keep the roller in those places for a few seconds until you feel the tightness dissipate. Foam roll as often as you'd like, especially after you exercise or before going to bed. Place a roller by your bed so you remember to do it.

DETOX YOUR SKINCARE PRODUCTS

Most personal care products are made up of some combination of 10,500 different chemical ingredients. In a day's time, the average individual uses nine personal care products that contain 126 of these unique ingredients. When used on your skin, some can strip away your skin's protective lining, clog pores, and decrease your skin's elasticity. But the effects are more than skin deep, as your skin absorbs them into your body where they can cause issues.

Researchers have found many of these ingredients in breast tumor tissue, human fat, and urine. Some of them have been shown to be carcinogenic, toxic to the reproductive system, or disruptive to the endocrine system, according to the Environmental Working Group (EWG). Avoid any product with these "dirty dozen," according to the David Suzuki Foundation: BHA and BHT; coal tar dyes (p-phenylenediamine and colors listed as "CI" followed by five digits); DEA, cocamide DEA, and lauramide DEA; dibutyl phthalate; formaldehyde-releasing preservatives; paraben, methylparaben, butylparaben, and propylparaben; parfum; PEGs; petrolatum; siloxanes; sodium laureth sulfate; and triclosan. Add hydroquinone to that list too.

For help finding clean cosmetics and skincare products, head to the EWG's Skin Deep Cosmetics Database (www.ewg.org/skindeep) or the Campaign for Safe Cosmetics (www.safecosmetics.org/get-the-facts/chemicals-of-concern/red-list/). Take it a step further by using the Leaping Bunny Program (www.leapingbunny.org) to search for products that don't use chemicals and don't test on animals.

GET MARRIED

Pairing up could lead to a lifetime of better health, even a longer life, as long as that marriage is flourishing. When you say "I do," you're signing on to more than just wedded bliss. Start with heart health. Numerous studies show that happily married individuals have better heart health, including better cholesterol levels and body mass indexes. In fact, one recent study even found such a strong link between marriage and protection against heart disease, stroke, and early death that it suggests marital status should be a risk factor for heart disease.

Happier marriages also lead to fewer severe diseases overall, less physical pain, and fewer hospitalizations. Even when you're trying to adopt a new healthy habit, your partner can help you not just start it but also maintain it. The icing on the cake (maybe even the one from your wedding if it's still in the freezer): married individuals, in general, tend to live longer than non-married folks.

CHOOSE A FLATTERING HAIRCUT

You can look younger—some stylists say by as much as ten years—just by choosing a different hairstyle. Everybody's different, of course, so you'll have to work with your stylist to figure out what's best for your hair, your face, and your lifestyle. But in general, here are a few tips to keep your face looking younger:

1. Opt for light layers that fall around your face, adding side-swept bangs.
2. Avoid bangs or bobs that are cut short or blunt; instead, wavy bobs and soft, wispy bangs work best.
3. Try a shag that looks messy and modern.
4. Get long hair cut into layers, because straight, long hair can appear to drag your face down.
5. Make sure your hair moves; hair that's too stiff looks old.
6. Choose loose waves over tight curls.

SPEND TIME IN GREEN SPACES EVERY DAY

Living near green space isn't only a boon for your happiness, it's also a life-promoting health booster. In recent years, as more people have moved into urban areas and new buildings have been constructed, the amount of green space in cities has dropped considerably. That's not a good thing for health, as the data has conclusively pointed to green space as being good for mind, body, and spirit. Without exposure to green space, it's possible you could become unhealthier.

What's the magic behind green space? For starters, it provides motivation to get out and move, which is why studies have shown that people who live near parks have lower body mass indexes than people who don't live by them. Folks are also more likely to meet recommended exercise guidelines and watch less TV when they live near green space. Depression, heart rate, and rates of violence drop while overall mental health and vitality improve. You might even gain a few years, as living near green space decreases the risk of death.

If you don't live near a green space, get creative. For instance, seek out a local park and take a walk there, eat lunch outside if your office is located near trees, or hop on your bike and go in search of green areas.

USE TAPE TO WARD OFF BROW WRINKLES

Furrowing your brow might be a daily habit you're not even aware of. Yet the more you frown, the more you wrinkle. That furrowing action is actually causing those wrinkles between your eyebrows and the bridge of your nose. The more you frown (or squint), the deeper those folds can become.

While you can't physically erase that frown line, you can get it professionally treated if you talk to a dermatologist. Or you can just reach for a piece of cellophane tape. Put that tape on your forehead when you're at home to remind you not to furrow your brow or squint. Repeated use of this simple trick will help you break the habit or, at the very least, make you more conscious about doing it.

AVOID CFL LIGHTBULBS

Sun exposure is the main cause of skin aging, but it's not the only light you should worry about. The surprising culprit you may never have considered? Compact fluorescent lamps (CFLs). Not sure if you have them? Check the box or bulb to see if it identifies the bulb as a CFL.

Although many companies are phasing out CFLs, you probably still have some in your lights at home or in your office. A study from Stony Brook University in Stony Brook, New York, revealed that defects in CFLs could allow UV radiation to leak out at levels high enough to cause the same kind of skin cell damage as sun exposure.

To get this exposure, though, you have to be close to the bulbs, which is why researchers recommend staying several feet away from these bulbs and making sure they're behind an additional glass cover (like a light fixture) and not bare.

CONNECT WITH YOUR COMMUNITY

Being part of a community actually builds your happiness and longevity muscles. In fact, connecting with others is so important that a Brigham Young University study found that being lonely and socially isolated is as big a threat to longevity as obesity. Other data shows that loneliness raises the risk of early death by as much as 30 percent.

Here's the surprise, though: loneliness and risk of death are stronger among individuals under sixty-five than those who are older. That echoes findings from a University of California, Berkeley, study in which twenty-year-olds, in spite of having larger social networks, reported feeling twice as lonely and isolated as people aged fifty to seventy.

You may already have a group of close friends, which is great—but you can also look to join groups of new people who are focused on issues or topics you're passionate about in life. For instance, if you love to read books, look for a book club, or if you're a fan of plant-based eating, see if there's a *Facebook* group that announces meet-ups with like-minded herbivores. Hang with them at least once a week.

DRINK PLENTY OF WATER

You already know how important water is to your overall health and appearance. Your skin is made up of 64 percent water, and if you don't drink the right amount of water regularly, you'll no doubt see the effects of dehydration, which can make wrinkles and fine lines look even more pronounced. Here's what you might not know: on average, women need 91 ounces a day, while men need 125 ounces, according to the National Academy of Medicine.

Fortunately, you don't have to meet this need by drinking water alone. You can also get water through foods like fruits and vegetables, as well as other beverages like coffee, tea, and juice. The Academy recommends getting 80 percent of your daily intake from water and other beverages (even if they're caffeinated), and the remaining 20 percent from food. Note that if you live in a hot climate or are super active, you might need more.

PUT BLUE LIGHT TO BED

A good night's sleep is a hallmark of good health and a younger appearance. But are you sabotaging your sleep with electronic devices? "Blue light" is emitted from almost all devices, including TVs, smartphones, tablets, and computers. When you use any of these at night, that blue light suppresses the release of sleep-promoting melatonin in your body. Because your body doesn't get signals to sleep, you stay awake longer than you normally would and have more trouble falling asleep.

Using these devices before bed also reduces the amount of rapid eye movement (REM) sleep you get. Your body cycles through five stages of sleep every night, including REM sleep. This is usually the stage when dreaming occurs, and it plays a role in memory, learning, and mood regulation.

You can use blue light–blocking glasses (your eye doc may sell them) or install screen-dimming apps like f.lux, SunsetScreen, or Iris. Even better? Stop using these devices thirty to sixty minutes before you crawl into bed. And don't put them near your bed or you could be tempted to use them in the middle of the night.

KEEP TURKEY NECK AT BAY WITH EXERCISES

No offense to turkeys, but turkey neck is an undesirable effect of aging. Father Time can cause skin, especially around the jowls, to lose its elasticity and sag. You might also notice that the skin on your neck is getting more thin and wrinkly, which you might not like.

To quell it, moisturize your neck and make sure you're using sunscreen on it every day, something you should start as soon as possible, as you may start seeing fine lines around your neck as early as age thirty-five. Also, if you're a smoker, quit, as cigarette toxins can worsen skin aging, even around your neck.

Another strategy? Do exercises for your neck, like a simple neck flexion and extension. Start by dropping your chin toward your neck and holding for a few seconds before returning to the start position. Keeping your shoulders down and back, lift your chin up toward the ceiling and hold for several seconds. Release to start and repeat several times.

WRINKLE-PROOF YOUR CHEST

Women, this hack's for you: décolleté or chest wrinkles. Chest wrinkles show up around and between the breasts and may start as fine lines that progress to deep wrinkles or folds. One common cause? The skin between your breasts being pushed together, and the more that happens, the more that skin creases. Chest skin not only has fewer oil glands, it's actually much thinner than other skin on your body. Sun exposure, having kids, and getting older are other common culprits.

To combat this, use a retinol-based cream at night and always use sunscreen on your chest. Check, too, that you're wearing the right bra size. Then sleep on your back, not your side. When you sleep on your side, chest skin will be pulled down by the weight of one breast. If you can't train yourself away from side sleeping, use a breast pillow. Just put the pillow between your breasts to support them and minimize movement of the chest skin, which could prevent lines and wrinkles. A breast pillow also helps ensure that you're not rubbing your breast against your arm, which can further tug at chest skin.

PROTECT YOUR HEARING

Everyone knows that some hearing loss comes with age. But is there anything you can do about it? Hearing loss affects one in three people between sixty-five and seventy-four years old. Once people turn seventy-five, nearly half of them have trouble hearing. It's inconvenient, upsetting, and even embarrassing not to be able to hear—but even worse, cognitive decline may actually occur 30 to 40 percent faster in older adults who have hearing loss versus those whose hearing is normal.

While this age-related hearing loss can't be prevented, there's another kind of hearing loss, one brought on by loud noise, that *can* be prevented. Because you can suffer from both, which makes your hearing even worse than if you just had one, it pays to protect those ears now, no matter how young you are. Consider this: between 1994 and 2006, hearing loss among American teens aged twelve to nineteen increased from 3.5 percent to 5.3 percent, largely because of listening to music through headphones. Experts believe this number will continue to rise.

Noise that's too loud and lasts for a long period (like lawn mowers, leaf blowers, firearms, snowmobiles, and music) damages sensory hair cells in your ears that help you hear. Once those cells are damaged, they can't be fixed.

That's why experts recommend following the 60/60 rule: keep the volume of devices under 60 percent (if you can't hear anything but your music, it's too loud), and limit listening to only sixty minutes at a time. If possible, opt for over-the-ear headphones, which are less likely to cause hearing loss from noise than earbuds.

PASS ON PROCESSED FOODS

Processed food accounts for over half of most Americans' diets. Processed foods are defined as those that have undergone numerous steps to be transformed from their original state to the food you're eating. Get this: 57.5 percent of the calories the average American eats every day comes from ultra-processed foods (think soft drinks, mass-produced packages of bread and buns, instant noodles and soups, reconstituted meat products, industrialized desserts, and packaged snacks). The remaining calories come from: 30.2 percent unprocessed or minimally processed foods (like pasta, beans, and vegetables), 9.3 percent from processed foods like cheese or vegetables in brine, and 2.9 percent from processed culinary ingredients like baking powder and baking soda, vinegar, and unsweetened baking chocolate.

So what's the harm? Plenty. Ultra-processed foods contain *eight* times the amount of added sugar as processed foods. You're also consuming more saturated fats and carbohydrates, even more chemical additives, and less of the good stuff like protein, fiber, potassium, magnesium, calcium, zinc, and vitamins A, C, D, and E. You'll then be at higher risk for chronic diseases like heart disease, cancer, and diabetes, and may even gain weight.

You'll see the effects on your skin too. Processed foods mess with the production of collagen and elastin, leading to a loss of elasticity and firmness in your skin. They can even make acne and rosacea worse.

One simple trick to escape this plague of processed foods: when you read labels, look for foods with fewer than five ingredients. Also, follow food journalist Michael Pollan's rule: "If it came from a plant, eat it; if it was made in a plant, don't."

EAT PRUNES FOR STRONG BONES

Brittle bones are an unfortunate part of aging, but there are lots of ways you can work to keep your bones strong as you get older. Bones grow the most through your twenties, which is when they achieve peak bone mass. That means that you've now probably already built your bone bank, as they say, and although you can certainly add a little to it as you age, your focus should be on maintaining it and not subtracting from it. Take too much from that bank and you could fall victim to osteopenia (a precursor to osteoporosis) or osteoporosis. Fractures become a greater possibility with those conditions. People at highest risk for osteoporosis and fractures are women over fifty. Once you have osteoporosis, you may shrink in stature and not be able to stand up straight, which could affect your daily function.

You can implement numerous strategies to help keep those bones strong, including participating in high-impact exercise like tennis or running, limiting your alcohol intake, not smoking, and doing strength training. Here's an even easier strategy: eat five dried plums (a.k.a. prunes) a day, which studies have shown can effectively help reverse and prevent bone loss.

TAKE A CAT NAP

Here's a health tip we can all get behind: a daily nap really could give your health a boost. One study showed that people with high blood pressure who took a mid-afternoon nap lowered their blood pressure for the next twenty-four hours and even used fewer blood pressure medications than non-nappers. And among Blue Zoners in Ikaria, Greece, midday breaks are a daily occurrence, leading Blue Zone researcher Dan Buettner to write that those who nap regularly might be able to cut their risk of dying from heart disease by up to 35 percent. Afternoon naps have also been shown to improve thinking and memory, enhance performance, decrease stress, and make you more alert, especially if you're coming off a bad night of sleep.

Napping comes with caveats, though. You could actually wake up groggier after your nap than before, something sleep experts call sleep inertia. Naps, especially if they're too long or taken too close to bedtime, can also interfere with your sleep at night, which can be problematic if you're already not sleeping well.

If you do want to nap, limit it to no more than thirty minutes or else you could suffer sleep inertia. Your best bet may simply be a quick power nap of ten minutes, which studies have found best reduces sleepiness and improves cognitive performance.

TRADE POTATO CHIPS FOR KALE CHIPS

Potato chips might be seen as somewhat healthy, given their first name. But because potatoes used in making chips have been so heavily processed that they've been stripped of any nutritional value, they are considered refined carbs, which can increase your odds of fine lines and wrinkles. They're also slathered in salt, which can cause skin inflammation.

If you must get your crispy, salty fix, try making kale chips at home. They might take a little getting used to, but they might also satisfy the same cravings—and give you a healthy dose of good-for-you nutrients. To make them, heat the oven to 350°F. Line a baking sheet with parchment paper or Silpat baking mat. After washing the kale, remove the stems and tear the leaves into large bite-sized pieces. Toss the kale with juice from half a lemon, ¼ cup nutritional yeast, and ½ teaspoon salt (optional). Massage kale gently and then spread on the prepared baking sheet so the kale isn't touching or overlapping. Bake 15 to 20 minutes until crisp and eat immediately.

KEEP TRACK OF YOUR FLEXIBILITY

Did you know that a loss of flexibility could signal heart issues? To measure your flexibility, do the sit and reach test. Although this test measures flexibility in your hamstrings and lower back, it can also indicate that you might have arterial stiffness. A study from *Heart and Circulatory Physiology* found that people over forty who had limited flexibility through their trunks may have arterial stiffness, a risk factor for heart disease. (The same didn't hold true for people under forty, by the way.)

To do a version of this test, place a yardstick on the floor, with a piece of tape perpendicular to the yardstick at the 15-inch mark. Sit on the floor with the yardstick between your legs, your heels touching the edge of the tape, and spread your feet about a foot apart. Moving slowly, reach your arms forward, keeping your palms down. Notice how far you stretch and release. Repeat and record your best reach. Use the following guide to score yourself:

Twenty-Six–Thirty-Five Years Old

- Above average: 20 inches
- Average: 19 inches
- Below average: 16 inches
- Well below average: 13 inches

Forty-Six–Fifty-Five Years Old

- Above average: 18 inches
- Average: 16 inches
- Below average: 14 inches
- Well below average: 10 inches

Thirty-Six–Forty-Five Years Old

- Above average: 19 inches
- Average: 17 inches
- Below average: 15 inches
- Well below average: 12 inches

Fifty-Six+ Years Old

- Above average: 17 inches
- Average: 15 inches
- Below average: 13 inches
- Well below average: 9 inches

If you're below average, mention this to your doctor. In the meantime, do stretching, yoga, and Pilates to improve future test results.

BANISH BROWN SPOTS

If your face looks like it has dirty or discolored spots on it, take heed: it's probably a condition called melasma. Although melasma is often brought on by pregnancy, women can get these brown or grayish brown spots even if they've never been pregnant. They typically develop after the age of thirty, and birth control pills are a common culprit. Often, though, they show up for no reason, and if you're spending time in the sun, they can look worse. They might even be triggered by being in hot conditions (like when you're doing hot yoga or spending time in a sauna or steam room).

Melasma's difficult to get rid of, but there are three things you can do to prevent it:

1. Avoid any exposure to hot or sunny environments.
2. Make sunscreen a priority, reapplying every two hours, and wear a hat when you're outside to offer additional protection.
3. Try a lightening cream with kojic acid, which helps lighten brown spots on the skin.

BUY ORGANIC

Organic foods may not be in everybody's budget, but if you can afford them, your skin—and overall health—will thank you. Non-organic foods are produced with synthetic fertilizers and pesticides, and non-organic poultry and livestock are treated with antibiotics and growth hormones. When you eat these foods, you're then ingesting all of those chemicals, which some dermatologists believe affects the skin, triggering things like acne (which can happen well past your teenage years). And of course, animal products alone, whether organic or not, can age the skin. But that's not all these chemicals do. One of the most alarming pesticides is glyphosate, the active ingredient in Roundup. One study found that levels of glyphosate in individuals over fifty who were tracked from 1993 to 1996 and 2014 to 2016 increased by 500 percent. While researchers are still teasing out the effects on human health, glyphosate was labeled a "probable human carcinogen" by the International Agency for Research on Cancer. Studies are also finding that it could alter the gut microbiome and possibly sexual development.

Organic foods, on the other hand, are produced via certain national standards, which don't allow the harmful chemicals that non-organic foods do. And although you might find trace elements of pesticides on organic foods, mainly from contamination by non-organic foods, you're greatly reducing your exposure to these chemicals by eating organic.

Whenever possible, cut your exposure to these chemicals by opting for organic foods, especially for meat and dairy products (although if you're a true anti-ager, you won't be eating those often anyway). Then try for organic when purchasing these produce picks, which the Environmental Working Group has called the Dirty Dozen because they contain the highest amounts of pesticides: strawberries, spinach, nectarines, apples, grapes, peaches, cherries, pears, tomatoes, celery, potatoes, and sweet bell peppers.

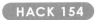

TAKE MAKEUP OFF BEFORE BED

Are you guilty of going to bed with your makeup on sometimes? That makeup, plus dirt, plus all the other junk that gets on your face in a day's time, can increase the population of free radicals on your face, which break down elastin and collagen. End result? Wrinkles.

Don't believe it? Check this out: when one woman stopped washing her face for an entire month (ugh, right?) and then just applied makeup every morning in an experiment run by a UK newspaper, dry skin made her wrinkles stand out more, her pores got bigger, and her skin became more uneven in spots. By not washing her makeup off every night, she aged herself biologically by a decade, creating deeper lines in wrinkles that already existed, making her skin look incredibly parched, creating more skin irritation, and causing her pores to become larger—which you typically see with aging skin.

No matter how tired or busy you are, always make time to take your makeup off before bed. For eye makeup, use something that's designed for the eyes, either a liquid or pre-moistened pad (if it feels too dry, run it under a faucet for a few seconds). Just make sure you don't tug or use firm pressure or you could create fine lines. For the rest of your face, use makeup remover wipes or cleansers. If you have a heavy layer of makeup, you may need to wipe or cleanse twice.

APPLY A FACE MASK AT HOME

Masks are part of every professional facial, and they're revered because they give skin a healthy glow while hydrating and minimizing wrinkles. While you can head to the spa, you can also use masks at home, either buying one or making your own. Masks have different purposes and formulations, so you need to know your skin type before you try anything at home.

- Clay or mud masks are best for dull skin and acne-prone skin.
- Gel masks can hydrate all types of skin but are especially beneficial for irritated skin.
- Want to hydrate or soften wrinkles and fine lines? Look for a cream or algae mask.
- For even more moisturizing benefits, choose a collagen mask.

You can also use oats. Just mix ¼ cup ground oats with 2 to 3 tablespoons water, stirring until the mixture is smooth and spreadable. Add more water or oats as necessary. After washing and patting your face dry, apply the oats to your face. Wait fifteen to twenty minutes and wash off with warm water. Then rinse with cold water.

CONSIDER COLLAGEN SUPPLEMENTS

Collagen is the main protein in numerous types of tissues in your body, including your skin, cartilage, and tendons. It gives strength and support to all of those structures, which is one reason it's crucial to your skin. Yet as you age, your collagen production decreases by as much as one to two percent a year, something that can start happening by the time you're thirty. The result? Fine lines, wrinkles, dull skin, and sagging.

When people have taken collagen supplements, though, the results have been positive. Studies have shown that collagen can improve skin hydration and skin elasticity and decrease deep wrinkles, mainly in women over thirty years old.

There hasn't been much official research on collagen supplements, so proceed with caution, especially because they can be expensive. If you do want to try it, you can buy it (in pill or powder form) or drink it—just skip collagen creams for your skin, which don't hold much merit. Most are sourced from animals (look for companies that get bones and tissues from antibiotic-free sources), but you can find vegan collagen supplements too. Experts suggest that 2.5 grams a day may be enough to get results. Also, remember that foods rich in vitamin C support your body's collagen production.

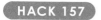

CHECK OUT A SUNSCREEN PILL

Believe it or not, there's a pill that could build your skin's sun defenses. It contains an extract from a fern that's native to Central and South America called Polypodium leucotomos. Studies have shown that supplements containing this fern, which is high in antioxidants and contains anti-inflammatory properties, may reduce harmful effects of UV radiation on DNA and collagen and help protect against sunburn. Some experts even recommend it for people with skin disorders that make them more sensitive to the sun. Note that these products don't need to be tested or approved by the FDA, which has issued some warnings about other sunscreen pills for misleading consumers. While products with this fern do have studies to back them, it's important to note that even if you decide to pop a pill with this ingredient, you still need to be diligent about wearing sunscreen.

You can find the oral supplement in most drugstores. Follow label instructions—some recommend taking one capsule a day at least sixty minutes before heading outside.

GO FOREST BATHING

The Japanese are famous for forest bathing, or what they call *shinrin-yoku*, and it could be one reason they're one of the world's longest-living populations.

What is forest bathing? Guides explain that it's the act of moving through a forest with no specific destination in mind. In other words, you're not trying to hike to that waterfall, you're simply enjoying your time among the trees. As you do this, your body's being doused in compounds called phytoncides, antimicrobial agents that trees bathe in to help combat things like bacteria and fungi that threaten them. You're breathing in these agents, too, which triggers the natural killer cells in your body that attack things like infected cells and tumorous growths. Studies have shown that forest bathing can also lower blood pressure and improve sleep. The upshot? A healthier, more vibrant you.

To try forest bathing, find a wooded area and just let your feet wander. Then at some point, sit for about thirty minutes (or as much time as you can) under a tree. Tune in to all of your senses and be conscious of what's going on around you.

BE A DAILY INSTAGRAMMER

Get your smartphone out now: it turns out that taking a daily photograph and posting it online could open the door to better well-being. As corny as this hack sounds, it comes from research in the United Kingdom that found that snapping a picture daily and then posting it online improved well-being in three ways:

1. It increased self-care.
2. It allowed people to interact with others, which was key for study participants who were retired and missed the office chatter.
3. It offered the opportunity for people to reminisce.

Other benefits included getting more activity (people actually went out of the house to look for cool places to take photographs) and feeling a greater sense of achievement, purpose, and competence. Study participants also felt more mindful.

Researchers call these daily pics an "active process of meaning-making." So *Instagram* or *Pinterest* away—it could be good for you!

EAT ALMONDS TO AVOID GRAY HAIR

You might be under the impression that your hair turns gray because it loses its natural pigments as you age. Not necessarily. Those grays are more the result of a build-up of peroxide that your hair follicles make. Your hair follicles also make an enzyme called catalase that essentially neutralizes that peroxide, keeping grays at bay.

Yet as you get older, your body not only produces less catalase, but the higher amount of peroxide also inhibits your body's production of catalase. End result? Gray hair, which can start as early as your thirties (generally thirty for men and thirty-five for women). Nearly half the population has 50 percent gray hair by the time they're fifty (experts call it the 50-50-50 rule). Smoking can also cause premature graying, especially before the age of thirty.

Whether you choose to embrace your grays, as many individuals are doing, or cover them is your choice. One survey found that gray hair can age women's appearance by six years, and men only three years. But you can help improve your body's production of catalase by eating certain foods—almonds in particular, which have been shown to increase catalase levels in the body. Just nosh a handful of unsalted almonds a day (avoid salty or flavored ones, which come with sodium, sugar, and extra calories). The bonus? You could also lower your cholesterol.

ADD SHINE TO DULLING HAIR

Got any apple cider vinegar in your pantry? It could be a simple solution to making dull, dry locks look younger. Your hair can lose its luster and dry out as you age, and the effects can start in your twenties. The good news is that apple cider vinegar is a natural way to restore shine to your locks. The vinegar is loaded with nutrients to help hair, and because of its slightly acidic level, it can help restore your hair's natural pH balance so that your hair shines again. It also helps remove dead skin cells and residue from sweat and hair care products, resulting in a shinier mane.

The recipe is simple: mix about 2 tablespoons of apple cider vinegar with 2 cups of water and pour it over your hair after you've washed it. Massage it into your scalp and then let it sit for several minutes before rinsing. Some people do this every week, but that depends on your hair, as it could do the opposite and make your hair even drier. To be on the safe side, start with every other week and see how your hair responds.

TEST FOR D-FICIENCY

Don't know your vitamin D level? Call your doc to get it checked.

Vitamin D is called the sunshine vitamin because your skin manufactures it when exposed to the sun. Foods also contain vitamin D, but it's tough to get the vitamin D you need from food alone. Plus, many people who live in northern latitudes where the sun isn't as strong all year are becoming deficient in vitamin D. A 2011 study indicated that almost 42 percent of Americans could be deficient.

That's not something to shrug off, as vitamin D deficiency has been associated with numerous chronic diseases like heart disease and cancer. Low blood levels of this fat-soluble vitamin have also been linked with high blood pressure, diabetes, fractures, asthma, and some autoimmune disorders.

The National Institutes of Health recommend that men and women aged nineteen to seventy get 600 international units (IU) of vitamin D daily, 800 IU if you're older than that. Although food sources of D are limited, you can find D in fatty fish like salmon and tuna, fortified ready-to-eat cereals, egg yolks, and light-exposed mushrooms.

You can also take vitamin D supplements, but before you do, get your levels tested through a 25-hydroxy vitamin D blood test with your doctor. The Vitamin D Council considers 0 to 30 ng/ml to be deficient, and sufficient to be somewhere between 40 and 80 ng/ml.

BOOST YOUR LASHES, NATURALLY

As you age, you expect your skin to wrinkle and your hair to gray, but who would have thought your eyelashes might suffer too? As it turns out, many people notice thinning lashes as they age.

One easy solution might be castor oil. While there's no science to prove that castor oil grows lashes, you can find tons of anecdotal evidence online to support its use. It's natural and doesn't come with side effects, and if nutrients like vitamin E in castor oil really do make those lashes thicken and grow, why not give it a try?

Start by washing your face and removing all makeup. Dip your fingertip or cotton swab into the oil and then apply it from the base to the ends of your eyelashes. Repeat several times a week, perhaps even at night so the oil has time to set. Just avoid getting that oil in your eyes, as it could irritate them.

If you're not getting results from this idea (some experts remain skeptical), ask your doc about Latisse, the only FDA-approved treatment to grow eyelashes. Although you'll need a prescription to get it, using it every night before bed has proven to be extremely effective.

STOP WEARING YOUR CELL PHONE

Wearing your cell phone on your body may be convenient, but your body could be absorbing lots of radiation as a result, possibly harming your health. Science is still determining the long-term consequences on human health from this radiation exposure, but there's enough data to suggest that using cell phones over a long period of time and in high amounts could affect human health. Some studies have shown heart rhythm disturbances and increases in blood cholesterol levels, and of course, there's always been the concern for cancer, which is why the International Agency for Research on Cancer labeled cell phones as possibly carcinogenic for humans.

Follow these tips to limit your exposure to the potentially harmful energy your cell phone emits:

- Keep your phone away from your body (so don't carry it in your bra or any pocket, especially if it's close to your heart).
- When your cell phone signal is weak, limit its use (your phone's energy output will surge then).
- Put your phone on airplane mode whenever possible.
- Always use a headset when talking on the phone.
- Avoid putting the phone by your bed at night.

ASSESS YOUR GUT HEALTH

The ancient Greek physician Hippocrates was right when he said, "all disease begins in the gut." Most of your immune system lies in your gut microbiome, an ecosystem in your intestines that houses trillions of bacteria and other organisms that directly affect your health. If things in your belly's garden are out of whack, your health will take a hit. Imbalances in the gut microbiome have been linked to obesity, diabetes, certain cancers, depression, rheumatoid arthritis, and Alzheimer's. Studies have also found a link between a healthy gut and healthy aging. In one study, people over one hundred (whom researchers called "ridiculously healthy") had a similar gut microbiome makeup as healthy thirty-year-olds. The takeaway? Keeping that gut healthy could lead to longevity.

Everybody's gut microbiome is different, but through a stool test—numerous companies now offer mail-in tests—a lab can determine what bacteria and how much of each kind lies in your gut, and make suggestions on how to make that gut even healthier. Changes might include eating more fiber, sleeping more, managing stress, and adding probiotics or fermented foods to your diet. Fortunately, simple changes can affect that gut quickly. For instance, gut health improves in as little as two weeks with a switch to a vegetarian diet.

HOP ON THE COQ10 BANDWAGON FOR SMOOTH SKIN

CoQ10 is a nutrient that your body makes, and it functions as an anti-oxidant, helping cells grow and protecting them from damage. Yet after you turn twenty-five, your levels of CoQ10 begin to decline. (Smoking can also cause CoQ10 levels to plummet.) By the time you hit eighty, those levels could be lower than what you were born with. The lack of CoQ10 as you age means your body won't be able to produce as much collagen and elastin, so you wind up with more wrinkling and skin sagging. (An aside: in people with issues like heart disease, Parkinson's, cancer, and diabetes, CoQ10 is often reported to be low, so you might ask your doc about taking a supplement, especially if you have heart disease, are taking statins, or are over forty.)

You can find CoQ10 in topical creams, and studies have shown that applying it to the skin can help diminish the appearance of wrinkles. It gives your skin valuable antioxidants and could aid in creating elastin and collagen.

WATCH YOUR TABLET PROPERLY

Got a tablet? Then you're probably suffering from tablet neck, too, which can age your body and your skin. You already know that looking down at a screen can create wrinkles in your skin. Worse? You're probably also using the tablet while lying propped on your side, and if you're pressing your hands on your face, over time that could tug at the skin, causing creasing and wrinkling. Not to mention, of course, that you flex your neck forward, which can cause postural issues. The worse your posture is, the older—and sometimes heavier—you can look. And then there's the neck and shoulder pain, which was higher in women than men in a recent study.

To avoid these issues, take a three-pronged approach, per study researchers:

1. Choose a chair with back support, which will also decrease pain.
2. Put your tablet on a stand, which will put you in a more upright posture.
3. Clip on a posture tracker device (a wearable device that tracks your posture) so that you get gentle alerts when you're slouching.

REDUCE EYE PUFFINESS

Just like your muscles, the tissues around your eyes weaken as you age. The fat that would have normally supported your eyes moves into your lower eyelids, hence the puffiness in those lids. You might even get fluid below your eyes, which makes the puffing worse, or dark circles under your eyes, which you may not like. Lack of sleep, genetic factors, allergies, smoking, and even fluid retention after a salty meal can up your risk of getting these bags.

When they strike, reach for two tea bags or two slices of cucumber, both of which contain antioxidants that may reduce inflammation and irritation. For tea, soak two caffeinated tea bags in warm water, then chill them in the fridge for a few minutes before placing them on your eyes for five minutes. Or place a slice of chilled cucumber over each eye for about five minutes.

SHUT OFF YOUR ROUTER AT NIGHT

You're exposed to tons of man-made electromagnetic fields (EMFs) on a daily basis. They come from microwaves, Wi-Fi, computers, cell phones, Bluetooth devices, and power lines. So what's the danger? Good question, and it's one that hasn't been answered conclusively. While many government organizations say that EMFs don't pose a danger to human health, the World Health Organization believes EMFs could be carcinogenic to humans. Some studies have also shown a link between EMFs and Alzheimer's.

While this doesn't mean you have to disconnect completely, at least turn your Wi-Fi router off every night. Those routers can be a significant source of EMFs, which means that if you're running that router twenty-four hours, you could be getting around-the-clock exposure, especially if you spend large quantities of time at home. It's even more critical if you have kids in the house, as EMFs pose the most danger to developing brains (it's one reason many schools in other countries have banned Wi-Fi). By turning that router off at night when you should be sleeping, you'll at least reduce some of your exposure to EMFs.

RID YOUR MOUTH OF BACTERIA WITH COCONUT OIL

Your smile is one of the first things people notice about you, and you will look younger if you keep your teeth white and your gums healthy. To help do that, you might want to try something called pulling, a therapy used in Ayurvedic medicine that essentially "pulls" bacteria and other harmful things from your teeth, gums, and tongue. Studies have found that it's one of the best natural ways to alleviate tooth decay (see hack #112 for why it's key to prevent tooth issues), and by using coconut oil, you're getting the benefit of its lauric acid, which is an antimicrobial.

It's easy to do: just swish 1 tablespoon of coconut oil in your mouth for fifteen to twenty minutes (start with just five minutes and progress if that's too much). When time's up, spit out the coconut oil and brush your teeth. Repeat daily if you'd like.

MOISTURIZE YOUR SKIN

As you age, your skin becomes thinner and drier. Skin dries through transepidermal water loss, which causes water to escape through your epidermis, the outer layer of skin, before evaporating. By applying moisturizer on your body and face, you either trap or replenish that moisture in the epidermis. In return, you reduce the appearance of wrinkles, especially on your face, and give your skin a healthy glow.

Your first consideration when choosing a moisturizer should be your skin type. If you have acne-prone or oily skin, a water-based moisturizer might be best (use it mainly on dry areas of your skin), while people with mature, sensitive, or dry skin might be better off with an oil-based moisturizer. If you have extremely dry skin, the American Academy of Dermatology recommends looking for a moisturizer with urea or lactic acid. You might even see a dermatologist if that dryness is excessive, as there are medications you can apply to the skin to help.

The best time to moisturize is after you've washed your face or showered. Do it within a few minutes of washing when your skin is slightly damp to get the best results.

Here's another easy hack: purchase a sunscreen with moisturizer, and you'll save not only money, but also time.

DITCH PLASTIC BOTTLES

Environmental impact of plastic bottles aside, they could be negatively affecting your health, and if you want to live to a ripe old age, it might be best to ditch the plastic bottle habit. Every time you sip from a plastic bottle, you're swallowing plastic. The World Health Organization recently discovered that among some of the most popular brands of bottled water, 90 percent contained small pieces of plastic, amounting to twice as many plastics in bottled water as tap water. Plastic also leaches harmful chemicals like phthalates, BPS, and BPA, which could increase your risk of conditions like heart disease, obesity, and certain cancers.

If possible, avoid single-use plastic bottles and instead use stainless steel or glass bottles and drink containers. If you must use a plastic bottle, choose one with a number one, two, four, or five and avoid those with numbers three, six, and seven, as they've been found to contain the most chemicals. Also, don't leave your water bottle in a hot car or in direct sunlight and don't ever microwave it. High heat can cause the plastic to leach even more chemicals into your drink.

AVOID MUFFIN TOP WITH HIGHER-WAISTED PANTS

Muffin top (or love handles, if you prefer) is that roll of fat that spills over your pants. It's a natural part of getting older. You typically gain fat as you age, especially around your midriff. Stress, lack of sleep, menopause, and a bad diet can all make muffin top worse. There are two types of fat: subcutaneous, the stuff that you can pinch, and visceral, which surrounds your organs. In most cases, that muffin top is the subcutaneous type. While visceral fat tends to respond quickly to changes, subcutaneous fat is stubborn. It's often the first type of fat you gain but the last you lose.

You can—and should—adopt a healthier diet so you're eating less sugar, avoiding refined carbohydrates (like white bread, white rice, and potato chips), and going easy on the alcohol. Trainers often like to say that good abs are made in the kitchen, not the gym, but that doesn't mean exercise doesn't have a place, and interval training and strength training are key.

But because subcutaneous fat can take time to lose, it might be easier to hide that muffin top in the meantime. Buy high-waisted bottoms that fit at your natural waist, a few inches below your rib cage and just north of your belly button. This look will smooth over bulges at your waistline.

DRY-BRUSH YOUR SKIN

Here's an easy hack to help you look younger: dry brush three to four times a week.

If you're not familiar with dry brushing, it's basically an exfoliation-plus-massage treatment rolled into one. You're simply moving a dry brush (or mitt) with hard bristles slowly over your body in circular motions. Lots of claims are associated with dry brushing, including getting rid of cellulite on your body—if only that were true!

The benefits of dry brushing aren't entirely clear because there aren't a lot of studies on it. But experts say that it can increase your body's blood flow and circulation, giving your skin a more youthful glow, and help remove dead skin cells. This can be especially helpful starting as early as your thirties, when your skin cells have a tougher time turning over and a build-up of those cells can make skin look dull.

One caution: don't brush too much or too vigorously or you could damage your skin. Instead, use gentle pressure as you move the brush in circular motions from your feet toward your heart. Look for a dry brush at any large drugstore.

FIGHT THIGH DIMPLES WITH STRENGTH TRAINING

It's estimated that 85 percent of women have cellulite (compared to only 10 percent of men), and starting as early as your thirties, it can show up as dimples on your thighs. You don't even have to be overweight to have cellulite. Blame not only hormones but also a slowing of collagen production, which can thin your skin and make cellulite more noticeable. Being less active can also increase these dimples.

Unfortunately, cellulite creams sold in drugstores don't really work. You can, though, try retinol-based creams to stimulate the production of collagen. Better yet, add lower-body strength exercises to your weekly routine, especially if you haven't seen thigh dimpling yet. Lower-body strength exercises like reverse lunges, lateral lunges, step-ups, single-leg deadlifts, and plié squats are some of the best preventive strategies, plus they can also help decrease some of that fat. Aim to do these exercises two or three times a week on non-consecutive days.

SPIT OUT THE GUM

Although activities like smoking and drinking through a straw are more associated with perioral wrinkles (those fine lines and wrinkles you get around your mouth), chronic gum chewing could also be a culprit. Every time you chew gum, you can exacerbate those wrinkles, either making them more visible or deepening them. Because your skin loses volume and elasticity as you age, those effects could increase over time.

In rare cases, gum chewing might even lead to masseter hypertrophy, a condition in which either or both of the masseter muscles in your jaw are enlarged, creating a jawline that's either square or uneven.

Easiest solution? Kick the habit entirely or chew in moderation, especially since sugarless gum does have some benefits, like improving memory, preventing cavities, quelling stress, and increasing alertness.

TAKE THE STAIRS

It's no secret that stair climbing is a cardio activity. Anybody who's traipsed to the top row of bleachers in a stadium knows this. Now add intensity to that stair climbing, do it for ten minutes straight (which includes warm-up and cool-down), and you've just improved your cardiorespiratory fitness, according to research from McMaster University in Ontario, Canada. It's a perfect exercise if you're short on time or lack access to a bona fide gym. Bonus? You can even do this on your lunch break.

Stair climbing after a meal could even help you lower blood sugar levels, especially if you have diabetes. In one study from BMJ Open Diabetes Research & Care, older adults who climbed stairs for three minutes at a time one hour and then two hours after a meal had lower post-meal blood sugar levels. It's also been shown to boost energy, maybe even more than coffee, and can build strength in the lower body.

Plus, climbing stairs now will help you avoid not being able to climb them in the future, since you'll not only keep your muscles strong, but you'll also keep your heart in shape. So shift some of your workout time to the stairs—climb them quickly to get a cardio boost or take two at a time to build muscle strength—and of course, always take the stairs whenever possible. One other trick? Adopt a no-elevator policy when traveling and use stairs whenever you're on a cruise ship or at a hotel.

WRITE IN A WORRY JOURNAL

Stress is no friend to aging. A whopping eight of ten Americans report feeling frequently stressed, the biggest stressors being kids and work, according to Gallup. The effects can show up instantly on your face with worry lines, and they become even more pronounced if you're not sleeping. And while you can't see inside your body, that stress could be wreaking havoc on your heart and other organs.

By keeping a worry journal, though, you dump your worries from your head onto a paper, and that alone can ease anxieties. You might also shift your perspective about your worries, even come up with solutions to some of them. To do it, take five minutes a day to write down some of your top worries and, if possible, a doable solution to each. Do this at any time during the day, although avoid doing it too close to bed or churning difficult thoughts could affect your sleep.

CARE FOR YOUR NAILS

Just like your facial skin, your nails change as you age. A little extra due diligence—and a daily biotin supplement—may be the solution. Nails actually get thicker as you age, plus they get more yellow and may break more. They might even grow slower, a change that's most noticeable after you turn forty, and develop ridges.

You can always schedule a pedicure or manicure—research indicates it could distract people from noticing aging signs on hands—but you'll need to do some home care in between appointments. Some simple strategies: always cut nails straight across, file snags with an emery board, wear shoes that fit your feet (consider alternating shoes so you never wear the same pair twice in a row), and most importantly, soak your feet if your nails are too thick to cut. Use a teaspoon of salt per pint of water, soaking them for five to ten minutes before trimming.

Some experts also recommend taking biotin for brittle nails. There's some evidence that taking 2.5 milligrams (mg) of biotin daily can thicken nails and reduce nail splitting.

AVOID METAL AVIATOR FRAMES

Sunglasses are key in preventing UV damage around your eyes—as long as you're not wearing aviator frames. While aviator frames certainly look cool and can be a fashion statement, they can pose a risk to the skin and increase the sun's harmful effects. How? The metal frames on those glasses actually reflect sunlight to your cheeks, which can cause them to burn. Over time, those burns can lead to wrinkling and dark spots.

So ditch the aviator frames completely, especially if you're heading to the beach or the slopes, but don't ditch wearing sunglasses. Just choose non-metal frames.

WATCH WHAT YOU EAT TO AVOID ACNE

Acne isn't just a teen thing. Between 40 and 55 percent of folks aged twenty to forty suffer from acne and oily skin. If you're a woman over twenty-five, the stats are even worse: 54 percent of you have some degree of facial acne. Numerous factors might be triggering adult acne, including work-related stress, diet, household worries, skin-irritating makeup, and, if you're a woman, those monthly hormonal fluctuations. And don't think you're off the hook if you never suffered from acne as a kid (lucky you!). You can still develop it in your thirties, forties, and fifties.

If there's any upside to acne, it's this: your skin might be aging slower. Research shows that wrinkles and skin thinning generally appear later in people who have had acne at some point in life. Acne sufferers tend to have longer telomeres than people who have never had acne, which could mean your body's cells are giving you better protection against aging.

That doesn't mean you want acne, though. To avoid it, change your diet by eliminating dairy products (especially those that are full-fat) and avoid high-glycemic foods, namely refined carbohydrates like white bread, baked goods, and cookies. Both of these food types can aggravate acne big-time, sending your skin into a downward spiral.

As for other ideas, the American Academy of Dermatology recommends checking hair and skincare products to make sure they're oil-free, non-acnegenic, and non-comedogenic. Use mild cleansers twice a day and apply a moisturizer daily.

FERMENT YOUR FOODS

Whether you make them or buy them, eating fermented foods regularly, if not daily, could be a lifesaver. What exactly are fermented foods, which, by the way, earned the number one spot among superfoods of 2018 in a *Today's Dietitian* survey? They're basically foods that have been produced in a way to encourage good bacteria to grow, something people have been doing for centuries. Examples include sauerkraut, kimchi, tempeh, kombucha, kefir, and miso.

Those fermented foods—and their accompanying bacteria—can offer your health a huge boost. They give your gut microbiome the food it needs to thrive, which means you could experience benefits like a stronger immune system, better digestion, and weight loss. Studies have also found that fermented veggies like kimchi can prevent cancer, lower cholesterol, and improve insulin sensitivity. Could they help you live longer? It's possible, as some of the longest-living folks in the world reportedly eat fermented foods daily.

DON'T SQUINT AT YOUR COMPUTER SCREEN

Ever heard of computer face? It's an emerging term, but it's essentially all of the squinting and frowning you do with your face (most of which you probably don't even notice) when you're using a computer or any screen. Do this repetitively day in and day out, and over time you'll age your skin prematurely. Everything from wrinkles and frown lines to deeper wrinkles can result. You could also develop turkey neck (see hack #144) just by looking down a lot.

To combat this, identify if you're straining to see the screen. If so, visit your optometrist to get your vision checked. Even more important, use good ergonomics when working at your computer so you don't have to squint and crinkle your face every time you look at the screen. First, position your monitor so that the top is about two to three inches above your eye level and you're not getting any glare from outdoor or indoor light (it helps to place computers at a right angle to windows and use blinds or curtains). Sit (or stand) about an arm's length away.

FORGIVE

Several years ago, researchers coined the phrase "forgive to live." Good advice, even if you just forgive one person. That phrase comes from a study of over 1,200 adults aged sixty-six and up, and it was one of the first to look at the connection between a long life and forgiveness. Researchers asked participants all sorts of questions about how likely they are to forgive somebody, whether they hold grudges, and if they're able to forgive themselves. Three years later, they checked back in with these folks and learned this: the people who could forgive only on conditional terms, meaning that they couldn't forgive until somebody had apologized to them first or promised not to do what they did anymore, died before others who weren't attached to conditional forgiveness. One point to note: some people in the study waited so long to get this apology that the person who "wronged" them passed away before offering it.

Other studies have found that forgiveness can have a positive effect on your heart and your immune system. You might even feel less anxiety and depression and greater happiness, all of which contribute to a longer life.

So don't wait until it's too late. Be the bigger person and forgive that person who's wronged you first. Even if you forgive only one person, you'll be closer to lessening the load on your heart—and eliminating a source of worry lines.

USE AN OATMEAL MASK ON OILY SKIN

Greasy skin isn't just an issue teens worry about. Oily skin might even plague you as an adult. The most common cause of oily skin in teens is changing hormones, and it's no different when you're an adult, especially if you're a woman. Even though your skin's oil production typically decreases as you age, it can ramp up as a result of going through menopause (that doesn't mean men can't get oily skin as they age, but it's more common in women). While some dermatologists say there's an upside to having oily skin—it gives you a glow and could help fend off environmental pollutants—it can also lead to acne, inflammation, and irritation.

To help get rid of some of the oil and other gunk on your skin, make a mask with ¼ cup rolled oats and 3 tablespoons honey. (If you don't use honey from bees, substitute a plant-based honey like Bee Free Honee.) Mix together and apply to face and neck, leaving it on for twenty-five minutes. Rinse with warm water.

HACK 186

GO NUTS! (BRAZILIAN, THAT IS)

A little nutrition 101: Brazil nuts contain some of the highest amounts of selenium, a nutrient that has anti-inflammatory and antioxidant properties. Selenium also has skin benefits—it can help prevent the breakdown of collagen, and some studies suggest that it can aid in protecting against age spots, sun damage, and skin cancer.

Although selenium plays many roles inside the body as well, perhaps its most important in terms of aging is that it helps the thyroid function. That's key as you age, because thyroid conditions increase as you grow up. Over 12 percent of Americans will develop thyroid issues at some point in life, according to the American Thyroid Association. One way to keep your thyroid in check is to eat enough selenium by popping one to four Brazil nuts a day.

Bonus? Just four Brazil nuts a month can help lower cholesterol, an effect that could last the next thirty days.

LOWER YOUR RESTING HEART RATE

When it comes to living longer and healthier, fitter folks have a leg-up. How do you know if you're one of them? Check your resting heart rate (RHR). RHR is your heart rate at rest, and it can provide valuable insight into your heart and other longevity factors. While you want it to beat harder during exercise, you don't want it working overtime when you're just doing normal activities, even resting. Some heart docs say, after all, that your heart can only tick so many times before it poops out.

A lower RHR means that you have a higher fitness level and less risk of heart woes, as your heart is able to pump more efficiently. Meanwhile, a higher RHR means your heart is pumping more, which will eventually affect its function and set you up for heart attack or early death. One study found that high RHR in men was associated with a higher number of circulating blood fats, increased weight, higher blood pressure, and increased risk for premature death.

To measure RHR, place two fingers on your wrist pulse while lying in bed in the morning and count for thirty seconds. Multiply by two to get your RHR. Normal RHR for adults is 60 to 100 beats per minute. If yours is on the high side, talk with your doc, as the previously mentioned study found that men with RHR of 81 to 90 had double the risk of early death, triple if it was higher than 90. You can lower RHR through exercise, even just one hour of high-intensity aerobic exercise a week. Check your RHR once or twice a week to see if it's improving (note that things like stress and medications can affect it).

LAUGH EVERY DAY

They say laughter is the best medicine, and laughing might also help you live longer! It's not just about putting you in a better mood. Other benefits include improving memory, decreasing stress and muscle tension, building social connections, and boosting your immune system. You can even burn calories—up to forty calories in just ten to fifteen minutes of laughing—and tone those ab muscles.

So get that laugh at least once a day. One study quoted a physician saying that he envisioned a day when doctors would prescribe fifteen to twenty minutes a day of laughing just as they prescribe thirty minutes of daily exercise. Hang around a funny friend as much as you can, watch a hilarious TV show or comedy routine, or pull up a belly-busting funny video on *YouTube*.

AVOID CREPEY SKIN

You want to eat crepes, not wear them. Yet as you age and your skin gets thinner, your skin can begin to "crepe," making you look like an elephant. Creping is different from wrinkling. While wrinkles form from repeated movement in one area on your skin, creping occurs when your thinning skin gets stretched and can't return to normal. Think crepe paper or elephant skin, and you know what this means. Crepey skin can happen anywhere on your body, although it's most common on your chest, knees, knuckles, and elbows. Blame crepey skin on the loss of collagen and elastin as you age, sun damage, less moisture in your skin, significant fat loss (even from aging), medications, and, for women, loss of hormones.

Fortunately, skin creping can be prevented and treated by using sunscreen daily, moisturizing your skin every day, and drinking enough water. Even better, apply topical creams with retinol daily. Retinol can increase elastin and collagen in your skin, giving it more structure.

MINIMIZE SPIDER VEINS WITH WARM COCONUT OIL

Check your legs: if you can easily see tiny veins below the surface of your skin, you've got spider veins.

Spider veins commonly appear on the calves, ankles, and thighs (although they can also appear on the hands, forearms, and face). Doctors aren't entirely sure what causes them, but they believe that weight gain, birth control pills, and hormonal changes can contribute, which is why they typically affect more women than men. Although your risk for spider veins increases after turning fifty, you can develop spider veins even as a young adult.

To combat them at home, warm some coconut oil and massage it into any affected areas for five to fifteen minutes once or twice a day. Coconut oil contains anti-inflammatories that should help diminish the appearance of spider veins.

EXFOLIATE YOUR HANDS

You exfoliate your face, so why not your hands? As you age, the skin on your hands gets duller, and dullness can lead to looking older. But if you exfoliate your hands, you remove dead cells that have accumulated on your skin, which restores a natural glow.

The secret ingredient you'll need is lemon juice. It not only brings that glow back to your hands, it also lightens age spots. You'll need ¾ cup of brown sugar, ¼ cup of olive oil, and 1 tablespoon of lemon juice (or use freshly squeezed lemon). Mix ingredients in a bowl and then place the scrub on your hands, all the way down to your wrists, massaging it softly into your skin. Rinse with cool water. Then moisturize and apply sunscreen. Notice how much brighter—and softer—your hands feel.

SOFTEN DRY FEET

Scaly, cracked feet will have you looking way older than your years. It's no secret that drier skin is part of the aging process, and nowhere is that more evident at times than your feet, which take a lot of pounding during a day (and your entire life). It's not just the daily wear and tear but also the diminishing supply of collagen that's making your feet so parched, increasing their vulnerability to cracking and drying.

Baking soda to the rescue! Believe it or not, baking soda can also help decrease inflammation, fight pain, increase circulation, and help heal some of that drying and cracking. Just add 1 cup of baking soda to 4 quarts of warm water and soak your tootsies for at least fifteen minutes. After, dry and moisturize your feet. Ah to spa feet!

REVERSE YELLOWING FINGERNAILS

Are your nails turning a little more yellow? Yellow nails have a lot of causes, including recent turmeric use, nail polish (especially if you're not giving nails time to "breathe" in between polishes), nail fungus, smoking, and age. Fortunately, though, you can decrease some of that yellowish tint with one of the three solutions:

1. **Lemon juice:** Pour a little lemon juice into a bowl and soak your fingertips in it for several minutes. Dip a soft toothbrush in the juice and gently scrub the color away.

2. **Hydrogen peroxide:** Mix $\frac{1}{3}$ cup of water with 3 capfuls of hydrogen peroxide and soak your nails for two minutes. Then, with a soft toothbrush, rub those nails with the mixture. After, use a cuticle oil, as hydrogen peroxide can be drying to the nails.

3. **Denture tablets:** Plop a few denture tablets into some warm water. Once dissolved, soak your nails for several minutes.

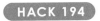

TREAT YELLOWING TOENAILS

Toenails can yellow for many of the same reasons that fingernails do, including excessive use of nail polish and aging. In some cases, though, the yellowing could be an indication of a fungal infection, so if the yellowing is accompanied by pain, swelling, bleeding, or a change in shape, call your doctor.

There are treatment options at home to make your toenails less yellow. While using a cough suppressant might seem odd, a study in the *Journal of the American Board of Family Medicine* found that Vicks VapoRub improves toenail yellowing in some folks, especially if it's caused by a fungus. The natural ingredients in Vicks appear to clear the infection in some people. Even if it doesn't work, it's worth a try, as it'll hydrate your nails at the very least. Just rub it on your toenails and then put socks on.

LET LAVENDER LULL YOU TO SLEEP

Studies show that lavender has sleep-promoting characteristics, helping you fall asleep a little easier by easing anxiety. In one study, people who slept in rooms where lavender oil was being diffused said their quality of sleep improved an average of 20 percent versus when they slept in a room where sweet almond oil was released. Even just sniffing lavender oil in two-minute intervals four times total before bed helped people get sounder sleep and wake up more energetic.

You can buy a premade lavender spray or make your own at home. In a 4-ounce spray bottle, mix together 20 drops of lavender essential oil and 1 tablespoon of isopropyl alcohol (or vodka). Fill the rest with water and shake. Each night, mist your pillows with this relaxing spray. No time to make this? Rub 2 or 3 drops of lavender oil on your palms (diluted according to instructions). Then cup your palms and inhale the scent before bed.

GREASE UP DRY SKIN ON YOUR JOINTS

Got a serious case of dry skin on your hands, elbows, or knees? Lather those dry spots with Crisco. It's a weird hack, for sure, but here's why it works: the soybean oil in the Crisco seeps deep into aging, parched skin, especially rough areas like your hands, elbows, and knees. Best part? It contains no scents and it's not made from chemicals, so it shouldn't bother sensitive skin.

Rub just a small amount on your dry spots, as a little can go a long way. If you're using it on your hands or feet, consider applying it at night and wearing gloves or socks over the Crisco to lock in the moisture even more (and avoid getting your sheets dirty). Then wash your hands and feet in the morning.

STOP USING HARSH SOAPS

Soap may be a bathing standard around the world, but for better facial skin, especially if you have sensitive skin or if you're prone to allergies, you'll ditch harsh bar soap on your face and choose a gentler cleanser. Many bar soaps, and even some liquid soaps, strip natural oils from your skin, which can lead to flaking, rough, and even itchy skin. That dryness can accentuate wrinkles and, in a weird twist of fate, cause your body to overproduce oil, which can clog your pores and lead to acne issues. There's also concern that bar soap wipes away the natural protective barrier on your skin, which keeps your skin hydrated and free from infection.

Not all soap is created equal, though, so do a little research and look for mild non-soap skin cleanser. It might use terms like *gentle, soothing,* or *ultra-calming.* Bonus? Look for one that's organic so you avoid harsh chemicals.

WEIGH YOURSELF DAILY

Love it or hate it, that scale could be an ally against weight gain. It's a fact: excess weight leads to a shorter life. Yet getting that weight off can be a daunting task. Unless, that is, you start stepping on the scale. Doing so daily could help shed unwanted pounds without any changes in diet.

When researchers put this to the test among college-aged women, those who weighed themselves daily not only lost body fat but also decreased body mass index versus those who didn't weigh in. The kicker? None of them were instructed to lose weight, which means that without any change in diet, they prevented weight gain and lost weight, something that typically doesn't happen in college.

That daily weigh-in simply gives you a check on how you're doing and could motivate you to eat better and exercise more. And if you see changes, it could prompt you to take action (some researchers suggest having a 5-pound window and acting if you go over that window). Just don't get hung up on the numbers. If you're becoming obsessed, check in less often (weekly) or dump the scale completely, especially if you've ever struggled with an eating disorder.

TRY ARGAN OIL ON YOUR FACE

Think oil's not good for facial skin? It is when you're using plant-based oils, many of which have gotten the thumbs-up in scientific studies for their skin-healing properties. One that won't break the bank? Argan oil.

Argan oil, which hails from Morocco, has earned fame for being good on all skin types. It's loaded with all of the nutrients your skin loves, including omega fatty acids, linoleic acids, and vitamin E. Because of its moisturizing properties, argan oil helps soothe dry spots on your skin and may even tighten sagging skin. It's been reported to give acne sufferers relief too. You can even try it on your brows and lashes to encourage them to grow.

If you want to give argan oil a shot, use it on skin that's slightly damp or on top of your regular moisturizer. You can also add a drop or two to your moisturizer. Don't worry that your skin will look like it's just been dragged through an oil slick, as argan oil is so lightweight that your skin will easily absorb it.

MAKE YOUR OWN FOOT SCRUB

Feet deserve the same royal treatment as your face, especially if you're battling dry, cracked, even callused skin. So show them some love with a scrub.

Feet are ultra-prone to drying because of all that you do on them and, depending on the weather, how exposed they are to the elements. By putting a scrub on them, you'll slough away rough and tough skin.

To make a soothing scrub for those feet, mix ¼ cup of brown sugar, 2 tablespoons of honey, 2 tablespoons of coconut oil, and 3 drops of peppermint essential oil. Using firm pressure, massage the scrub into your feet. Rinse with warm water and dry feet before moisturizing them. If you've got leftover scrub, store it in a closed container and use it within the next month.

HAVE ED CHECKED OUT

Men, if you're struggling with erectile dysfunction (ED), call your doc and get your heart checked. ED affects about 5 percent of men who are forty, but as men age, that number increases to roughly 15 percent of men around age seventy. The consequence isn't just poor performance in bed, though. Studies have found that ED may be one of the first signs of heart disease or a cardiac event, something most men are unaware of.

When something interferes with blood flow to the penis, you're unable to get an erection, and one of the causes could be clogging of those blood vessels. Because the vessels going to the penis clog earlier than those around the heart, ED can be an early warning sign of heart issues, and given that heart disease remains men's number one killer, it requires attention.

Call your doctor if you are having trouble and ask to have your heart checked. You can also take action by quitting smoking, logging more exercise, and losing weight.

EXFOLIATE YOUR LIPS

Lips need as much attention as your face to quell the effects of aging. As you age, your lips generally start thinning and can start losing their color in your thirties and forties, which can age your appearance. Lips get smaller for the same reason that your face is showing its age: your skin is losing collagen. Without enough collagen, your skin loses its structure, which your lips need to maintain their firmness and shape. Loss of collagen production also affects elastin and hyaluronic acid, both of which your skin needs to maintain its structure. Some experts have even suggested that because your face may be losing bone density as you age, thus giving you a more sunken appearance, lips can look thinner.

So what do you do? First, wear lip balm or ointment with SPF every day. Sun damage can slow collagen production. And if you're a smoker, quit, as lip thinning can be one of the many consequences of smoking. Stay hydrated, as lack of moisture can make lips dehydrated, and try to avoid licking your lips when they're dry, which will only make dryness worse.

But here's a hack you might not have heard: exfoliate lips at least once a week. Mix equal parts brown or white sugar with coconut or olive oil, or try a coffee scrub by mixing a tablespoon of coffee grounds with ½ tablespoon of olive oil. Gently massage onto your lips, rinse, and moisturize.

ONLY RUB YOUR EYES GENTLY

Guilty of aggressively rubbing your eyes every day? Join the club. Everybody rubs their eyes, especially first thing in the morning or during allergy season. Yet if you're using brute force to do this, you're damaging that already delicate skin and giving wrinkles a fertile breeding ground. That skin around your eyes is some of the thinnest on your body, and when you rub it, especially when you do so aggressively, you're wearing out that skin even more, making it more likely that wrinkles will develop, and it could increase the appearance of dark circles under your eyes.

It's impossible *never* to rub your eyes. But do be more aware of how you're rubbing them and use a gentler touch. And when you have to itch that eye, place only one or two fingers on the itchy spot and use as little pressure as possible.

DON'T REST YOUR HEAD IN YOUR HANDS

Your hands are a natural rest for your head, especially when you're lying on the floor or leaning on a counter. Yet doing this repeatedly has two big downsides. First, it could introduce your face to germs and bacteria, which could trigger an episode of acne. But worse, especially if you're worried about aging in your face, it can put pressure on your skin—much like a cotton pillowcase might do when you're sleeping—and eventually create lines and wrinkles.

It's a tough habit to break, especially given that the average person touches his or her face 3.6 times per hour every day, and you may not even notice how much you're doing it. But if you want to ward off wrinkles, you'll become aware of how often you're doing this and work to break the habit. When you notice yourself doing it, readjust your posture and find a different way to relax.

GROW PLANTS IN YOUR HOME

Go buy a new plant for your house. While extending your life, it could be a skin-saver too. If you read hack #243, you know that indoor air is often more polluted than outdoor air, and those pollutants can do damage to the skin by increasing wrinkling and age spots.

Yet studies done by NASA have found that placing plants indoors can improve indoor air quality. In just a matter of twenty-four hours, they can clear the air of harmful toxins like those found in formaldehyde, cigarette smoke, and household chemicals. Another bonus? Having plants indoors can also reduce your risk of death, in part because of the mental health benefits you gain.

Some of the best indoor plants (many of which are super easy to take care of) for improving air quality include mums, Gerbera daisies, peace lilies, dracaena, English ivy, snake plant, and ficus, according to the *Farmers' Almanac*.

GIVE YOUR BROWS A BOOST

Vanishing eyebrows could use a helping hand—or two—in the form of easy DIY treatments that rely on castor and olive oils. You might not give your eyebrows much thought unless you're plucking them. Yet as you age, those brows not only become coarser and—gulp—gray, they also become thinner.

Fuller brows can subtract years from your face, which is where plant-based oils may be of help. Castor oil and olive oil contain nutrients that can encourage hair growth. Using them is easy. Just rub whichever one you prefer into your brows each night before going to bed and then rinse in the morning. Do this daily to maximize results.

ADD SEA PLANTS TO YOUR SKINCARE REGIMEN

Seaweed isn't just a superfood, it's also a super anti-ager, which is why you should consider adding seaweed-based skincare products to your daily routine. Numerous companies have been sourcing ingredients from the sea for years, and many dermatologists believe they can help slow the signs of aging. Plants from the sea have to undergo harsh and changing conditions, which increases their antioxidant properties, including vitamins B and C. Seaweed is loaded with proteins like amino acids, and minerals like zinc and magnesium, all of which are beneficial to your skin. They're also humectants, meaning that they can draw moisture to your skin. As a result, they're especially potent against the formation of wrinkles on your skin and may also help protect your skin against sun damage, moisturize your skin, and increase your skin's production of collagen.

Next time you're shopping for skincare products, especially moisturizers and masks, look for those that contain seaweed, algae, or chlorella.

PAMPER THINNING TRESSES

If your mane isn't as thick as it used to be, take heart: a simple scalp massage can help build that hair. Everybody, no matter their age, loses hair daily—to the tune of about 100 to 150 strands. While you don't necessarily lose *more* hair as you age, your hair does lose volume because your hair strands are becoming thinner and finer. Thinning hair can become more pronounced over time and tougher to hide, especially because your hair is one of the first things people notice about you.

If you think you might be losing more than usual on a regular basis, check in with your doctor, as it could indicate a health issue. However, if it's just thinning because of age, here's a simple trick to stimulate that growth: massage your scalp. If you do this for four minutes a day, you could increase the thickness of your hair in twenty-four weeks. Adding a little coconut oil to your massage could make that hair even stronger.

DRAW A BEER BATH TO BRIGHTEN SKIN

While science says that drinking beer might make you happy, soaking in it could make you look younger.

Beer baths are nothing new in countries like the Czech Republic and Germany, and legend has it that they reach as far back as the ancient Romans and Egyptians. But in the States, beer baths are just gaining traction at numerous spas, and there's good reason to say cheers to that. The combo of hops, which are loaded with antioxidants, and brewer's yeast, which has B vitamins that brighten and soothe skin, makes a beer bath the perfect antidote for aging skin. Even better? If you've got acne, that brewer's yeast could kill acne-causing bacteria.

Fortunately, you don't have to travel to a spa or a different country to get the benefits. Make your own beer bath at home by pouring a can of beer—any kind will do—in your tub full of water.

LIMIT SCREEN TIME

Digital devices are such a large part of everyday life that it would be hard to live without them. And while they do have benefits, there are some downsides. Digital devices not only interrupt sleep, they also make people more sedentary, which leads to weight gain. They can increase loneliness, depression, stress, and anxiety, and decrease personal connections with other people. They can even damage eyesight, interfere with focus and productivity, and lower levels of empathy.

So set a rule that you'll only allow two hours max of non-work (or non-school) time on them a day (doing this will also make you a good role model if you have young kids, most of whom use screens too much). Anything over that is excessive. Some tips for sticking to this new habit: avoid checking devices thirty to sixty minutes before going to bed and after waking up, put away devices at meals, and declare your bedroom a no-device zone.

GIVE UP MODERN CONVENIENCES ONCE IN A WHILE

Crazy as this hack sounds, getting rid of things that make your life easier could extend your life. When you look at some of the longest-living, slimmest folks in the world, they don't do structured workouts in fancy gyms. Yet they do move a lot during the day, largely because they don't have modern-day conveniences like garage door openers, TV remotes (if they even have TV, that is!), and dishwashers, all of which have factored movement out of your daily life. One researcher has even concluded that all of these modern-day conveniences make you burn 111 fewer calories per day, which amounts to a whopping 10 pounds of extra weight a year.

So change that by doing more things by hand when you have the time and energy. For instance, mash potatoes with a hand-masher versus a mixer, walk your next round of nine holes versus riding in a cart, or use a push mower rather than a riding mower. These simple swaps can improve your fitness level and extend your life.

AVOID EXERCISE-INDUCED BREAST SAGGING

Women, make sure you're wearing a supportive, properly fitted sports bra. Otherwise, you could fall victim to premature boob sagging. High-impact exercises like running are great for slimming that waistline, strengthening your heart, and boosting bone density, yet those activities may also cause premature boob sagging by breaking down collagen in your breasts, which leads to sagging. You should obviously continue exercising, since that brings you myriad health benefits, but if you want to avoid breast sagging, be sure to invest in a high-quality sports bra as well.

To choose the best sports bra for you, consider the types of activities you do most and your body type. Are you doing lots of bouncing? If so, you'll need a sports bra that can support that bounce. Then, consider which straps feel best for your size and shape—wide shoulder straps or a racerback. As you're trying on sports bras, do the activity you're purchasing the sports bra for. For instance, if you're a runner, run in place in the dressing room to determine how supportive the bra is. Then take care when washing it: wash it in cold water and line dry it (the heat of the dryer could weaken stretchy fabric). And replace your sports bras regularly—some experts recommend once a year.

GET RID OF UNWANTED FACIAL HAIR

Many women find themselves growing unwanted facial hair as they age. This hair growth in women is most often visible around the mouth and chin. For some women, the hair growth can be excessive—a condition called hirsutism—but even if it doesn't progress that far, extra facial hair can damage self-esteem. Hormone imbalances are often to blame, and although excess hair can start shortly after puberty in women, it can also hit premenopausal women and continue for several years after menopause.

If you'd like to banish hair on your chin or upper lip, try an at-home wax. Mix 1 tablespoon of brown or white sugar with 1 tablespoon of raw honey and 1 tablespoon of water. Microwave the mixture for about thirty seconds until it's bubbly and a little brown. Let the mixture cool. Using a spatula, apply the wax to the facial hair you want to remove. Now take a thin cloth strip and press it smoothly over the area in the direction of your facial hair growth. Then quickly pull the strip off your face in the opposite direction of that hair growth. Repeat again on other places if needed.

APPLY MOISTURIZER WITH UPWARD, CIRCULAR MOTIONS

Facial skin starts to sag over time. The obvious reason is because of changes in your skin's structures, including your bone, fat, and tissue. Your skin is also losing elastin and collagen, both of which help keep your skin firm. These age-related changes lead to that sagging, but there are other factors, too, many of which you have control over, including sun exposure, smoking, your sleeping position, and your facial expressions. Just don't forget gravity, which literally pulls everything down.

You obviously can't fight that gravitational pull, but you can avoid making it worse by using upward or circular motions whenever you're applying product to your face. Many people are guilty of rubbing downward when they wash their face or apply moisturizer. By doing this, you're pulling the skin down even more. Instead, use an upward, circular motion with a light touch.

SIP RED WINE

Wind down with red wine and you'll be in good company: some of the longest-living folks in the world enjoy a glass of red wine regularly, often daily.

Red wine contains a compound called resveratrol, which is found in grapes (you can also get it from peanuts, cranberries, blueberries, dark chocolate, and pistachios). Resveratrol is loaded with antioxidants, and studies suggest that it can help lower blood pressure, protect the brain, help ward off certain cancers, and may have anti-aging benefits. Plus, red wine may help your gut microbiome.

While it's too early to suggest taking a resveratrol supplement, some experts agree that it's okay to drink a glass of red wine every now and then, perhaps even daily. (Sorry, there's not enough evidence to suggest *starting* if you don't drink already.) If possible, choose wine that's been produced organically or biodynamically; otherwise, you could be sipping down chemicals like pesticides and fertilizers.

KNOW YOUR BRA SIZE

Here's a surprise for women: wearing the wrong size bra could make you look older, even heavier, which is why it's time to get a professional fitting. Your breasts are in constant flux as you age. Losing or gaining weight, pregnancy, and your monthly cycle can all cause fluctuations in breast size. Because your body is producing less collagen as you get older, your breasts can also start sagging. All of this means you may need to switch bra sizes throughout the years.

Wearing the wrong bra size isn't only uncomfortable, it can also cause your breasts to sag, especially if you have a bigger chest. Saggy breasts pull on the skin, which makes the drooping—and possibly wrinkling—worse. Not only do you look older then, you also look heavier.

That's why it's worth a trip to a bra specialist to get properly fitted. You can find such a specialist in department stores or specialty bra shops. In general, though, your breasts shouldn't spill over the cups (if so, the bra is too small), and you shouldn't see any wrinkling or gapping at the top (that means the bra is too big). The perfect fit is one that holds and supports your breasts. Any bra should also allow about an inch between your breasts. If you're wearing underwire, make sure it rests against your body.

TRY MATCHA

Matcha is famous for its green glow (thanks to its chlorophyll content) and celebrity enthusiasts. Because it's made from dried and crushed tea leaves, matcha contains a significantly higher amount of antioxidants and other nutrients than other teas, like white or green. One antioxidant of note? The catechin levels. One study found that it contains three times more epigallocatechin gallate (EGCG), a powerful health-promoting antioxidant, than other green tea, and 137 times more EGCG than China Green Tips green tea.

That may explain why matcha has been associated with helping prevent certain cancers, promoting "alert calmness" (thanks also to its mix of caffeine and another compound called L-theanine), and improving heart health.

Matcha also has beneficial effects for your skin, working against aging by protecting the skin from UV damage, pollution, and other irritants. And when used on your skin, matcha may even combat wrinkles, dark circles, and skin inflammation. Here are two ways to use matcha:

1. Make a matcha latte: Whisk ½ teaspoon cooking-grade matcha into an 8-ounce mug. Add 1 tablespoon hot water and mix until it forms a paste free of lumps. Add 6 ounces coconut or almond milk and mix or whisk (or use an electric hand frother). Add sweetener of your choice.

2. Make a matcha face mask: Combine 1 teaspoon cooking-grade matcha with ½ teaspoon (or more if you prefer) raw honey. Slather it on your face and leave on for fifteen minutes. Rinse with warm water.

MINIMIZE KNEE WRINKLES

Wrinkles don't just appear on your face and hands—your knees may wrinkle too. It only makes sense, given how much your knee skin moves in a lifetime. That stretching, plus the loss of collagen and muscle mass as you age, makes knees vulnerable to looking crinklier, weathered, and leathered.

One easy way to improve your knees' appearance is to moisturize them daily. If possible, apply the moisturizer at night and then pull long socks around your knees to lock in the moisture as you sleep. Exfoliate them several times a week, too, so dead skin cells will be sloughed off.

Even better, add a squat to your fitness routine (or if you belong to a gym and a machine is preferable, choose leg extensions). Muscle loss could be one reason you're seeing these wrinkles. Doing lower-body strength exercises (like squats) that target muscles around your kneecap can help rebuild muscle in that knee area, which should help improve that sagging and even prevent future sagging. Stand with your feet shoulder-width apart. Keeping your weight in your heels, lower until your thighs are almost parallel to the floor—if you can go lower, even below your knees, do so, as you'll target the quadriceps. Release to start and repeat. Do twelve to fifteen reps at least two times a week.

SOAK IN A SALT BATH

Here's a relaxing way to restore aging skin: take a salt bath. The proof: researchers asked folks to submerge one arm for fifteen minutes in water containing some salt from the Dead Sea while soaking the other arm in tap water. They then compared the skin of both arms and found that the salt-treated skin was more hydrated than the other. The salt also lessened skin roughness and redness. Other studies have found that Dead Sea salts can even protect against UV radiation. What's the magic? Dead Sea salt is rich in magnesium, which not only exfoliates skin but also helps bring moisture deep within the skin so you're being moisturized from the inside out.

Can't get to the Dead Sea anytime soon? Just visit the store and pick up some Epsom salt, which is also a magnesium salt. Add 2 cups of the salt to warm bath water and soak for a minimum of twelve minutes, repeating several times a week.

DON'T OVEREAT

Mindless eating can lead to serious weight gain. To remedy this, follow the Japanese philosophy of eating until you're 80 percent full by practicing "hara hachi bu."

Weight often becomes tougher to manage as you age, especially if you're not taking steps to prevent it, and wearing that weight is a visible sign of an aging body. That may be why society, in general, tends to view thinner people as younger and heavier folks as older.

One problem that often results in weight issues is mindless eating. People who eat without paying attention to what or how much they're eating may end up eating past the point of fullness. Those daily eating episodes then begin showing up on the scale.

In the Japanese culture, though, people practice something called "hara hachi bu," which essentially means eating until you're about 80 percent full. That's about the time when you feel some pressure on your stomach. Once you feel that pressure, it's time to stop eating. You can make your mealtime experience last longer by taking smaller bites, chewing thoughtfully, and savoring the various flavors of the food you're eating.

STOP USING VEGETABLE OILS

People sometimes think that vegetable oils like soybean, sunflower, saf-flower, canola, and corn are healthier than butter. But unfortunately, they're all bad for you.

Vegetable oils are highly processed foods (and you already know how bad those are for you), and they contain high amounts of omega-6 fatty acids, which cause inflammation in the body. The more omega-6 foods you eat, the more inflammation you'll create, which could lead to diseases like heart disease, diabetes, cancer, and depression. They're also loaded with trans-fat, which has also been associated with chronic disease.

If you want to be truly healthy from the inside out, you'll make a complete break with vegetable oils. If you must use oils, many nutrition experts say using extra-virgin cold-pressed olive oil, even better if it's organic, is okay. But if you want to be truly healthy from the inside out, you'll make a complete break with vegetable oils.

Surprisingly, cooking and baking without oil is easier than you think. To cook without oil when stir-frying or sautéing, use nonstick cookware and replace oil with water or vegetable broth, adding a few tablespoons at a time and stirring frequently so your food doesn't burn. Want to swap out oil in baked goods? Try mashed bananas or unsweetened applesauce.

TIGHTEN YOUR PORES WITH ARTICHOKES

It's true: the pores on your face really do get bigger as you age. Blame the breakdown of collagen and elastin in your skin and the downward pull of gravity for causing pores to stretch open, something that can happen as early as your twenties. Those pores then look bigger, which can make you look older. One survey found that almost 75 percent of women reported looking younger with smaller pores.

Here's a food hack that can help, though: artichokes. They contain a compound called cynaropicrin, which minimizes the appearance of pores. You can eat them if you like, but you can also put them right on your skin. Make a mask with either a well-cooked artichoke hearts or a can of artichoke hearts in water. Mash the artichokes first and then combine 2 teaspoons of olive oil and 1 teaspoon of fresh lemon juice or vinegar. Stir until you have a paste and then apply to your face and skin, letting it sit for ten to fifteen minutes. Rinse first with warm water and then cold water to really tighten those pores.

ADD SEEDS TO YOUR DIET

Seeds have made their way into mainstream health foods like salads and grain dishes, and rightfully so. Seeds like flax, chia, hemp, sesame, and pumpkin are superstars of nutrition. They're rich sources of fiber, protein, and antioxidants, and each one comes with unique properties and benefits. Take, for instance, flax, chia, and hemp, which are high in omega-3 fatty acids, one reason they're so beneficial for vegetarians and vegans. And while flaxseed may lower blood pressure and cholesterol and reduce cancer risk, chia seeds are effective at cutting your risk of heart disease. Meanwhile, sesame seeds can help reduce inflammation in your body and cut oxidative stress, while pumpkin seeds can aid heart health.

That's why it's best to eat a variety of seeds, adding them to at least one meal a day. Try, for instance, making a breakfast pudding with chia seeds: soak 1 tablespoon of chia seeds in your favorite non-dairy milk for a few minutes before adding ⅓ cup of rolled oats and 1 tablespoon of cacao nibs; place in the fridge overnight and enjoy the two-serving breakfast in the morning, sweetening with maple syrup. You can also toss flaxseed in your salad. One note about flaxseed: the outer shell of the seed is hard to digest, which is why it's best to grind flaxseeds before using them. Just don't grind too many at once, as they will go rancid over time, and make sure to store them in a fridge.

MEASURE YOUR MILE SPEED

The fitter you are, the longer you'll live. One way to test your fitness? See how fast you can run a mile. What can a single mile run tell you? Plenty, including how healthy your heart is. Your fitness, after all, is a measure of your cardiovascular fitness. One study on over 66,000 individuals found that how fast you run that mile is a good predictor of your risk of having a heart attack or stroke. For comparison's sake, a fifty-five-year-old man who needed fifteen minutes to run a mile had a 30 percent lifetime risk of developing heart disease, versus a fifty-five-year-old man whose heart disease risk over a lifetime was less than 10 percent by running a mile in eight minutes.

You can easily do the test at home by running a mile on a treadmill or track and logging your time. If you can't run or haven't been doing much exercise, just use the one-mile test to gauge your aerobic fitness. Just mark off a mile (a school track is ideal) and walk that mile as fast as you can. Then use the following chart developed by the Cooper Institute:

Under Age Forty
- Excellent: 13:30 minutes or fewer
- Good: 13:31–16:00 minutes
- Average: 16:01–18:30 minutes

Over Age Forty
- Excellent: 14:30 minutes or fewer
- Good: 14:31–17:00 minutes
- Average: 17:01–19:30 minutes

If your number isn't what you'd like it to be, try to improve it (so test yourself again in a few weeks) by exercising regularly, doing high-intensity work at least once a week, and cross training.

SIP YOUR GREENS

Juicing is all the rage in healthy eating these days, but among them, green juices go to the top of the nutrient-packed list. Green juices are usually loaded with spinach or kale, celery, cucumber, spirulina, and parsley, and these foods are powerhouses in terms of nutrition for your skin (and your whole body, of course). For instance, the omega fatty acids in spinach can create healthy, glowing skin, while cucumbers and celery increase hydration in the skin.

Many skincare experts recommend drinking at least one green juice a day for glowing skin, and it's wise advice, especially if you're struggling to eat the greens (or any fruits and veggies, for that matter) you need. One note: juicing strips the fiber from fruits and veggies, so you'll be missing that valuable nutrient.

Also, beware of the green juices you can buy in bottles on store shelves. A recent report from *Consumer Reports* revealed that many of these drinks are high in sodium and sugar and don't actually contain many vegetables. If you do want to buy a green juice, check to be sure that it contains lots of veggies, little fruit juice, and as little sugar and sodium as possible.

Better yet, make your own at home so you can control what goes into it. Blend 2 cups chopped spinach, 1 apple (core and chop first), 1 stalk celery, fresh lime or lemon juice to taste, and ¾ cup water. Enjoy!

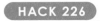

EMBRACE PROBIOTICS

Pop a daily probiotic, and you'll not only keep your microbiome happy, you'll also keep your skin glowing. You can get probiotics from fermented food, but you'd be wise to add a supplement to your daily routine, too, especially if you're not eating fermented food every day or follow the standard American diet (this diet causes bad, unhealthy bacteria to proliferate). That probiotic feeds your gut bacteria, which runs the show when it comes to your health. With the right bacteria in your gut, your health will thrive, making it easier to age with grace. Building a bigger colony of healthy bacteria can also clear up skin issues like acne. Data even suggests that probiotics can help either prevent or alleviate the consequences of UV-induced skin damage.

Probiotic supplements can be hard to shop for because they're not customized to your gut's individual needs. But there are a few guidelines you can follow. Choose one that has a high number of live organisms (so anywhere from five to thirty billion per capsule or teaspoon of powder). Look, too, for strains like Bifidobacteria and Lactobacillus. And always make sure you're taking a probiotic if you're ever put on antibiotics, which can wipe out good gut bacteria in no time.

Another strategy? Look for skincare that contains probiotics, as they could help reduce inflammation from conditions like acne and rosacea.

JUMP!

Jumping on a mini trampoline might sound like child's play, but this bouncing could be an effective, joint-friendly way to get the exercise you need—and then some. "Rebounding" classes have been around for several years, and there's good reason to give them a try. Rebounding is a joint-friendly activity, which means that if you're suffering any type of joint pain, it's worth asking your doctor if rebounding could help. Studies show that when overweight women did rebounding for twelve weeks, they improved blood pressure, increased cardiovascular fitness, and lost body weight and fat. Rebounding can also help lower cholesterol, improve coordination, and help fight fatigue. And it's so much fun that you might have an easier time sticking with an exercise program.

You can take rebounding classes at health clubs or buy a rebounder for use at home. When shopping for a rebounder, make sure it can accommodate your weight and has a colored ring around its edge to help your peripheral vision. Also, look for a trampoline that comes with an accompanying routine and safety instructions so you can learn what to do (and not do) on it. After that, the possibilities are endless, as you can do cardio, strength, and flexibility work on a rebounder.

SOFTEN ELBOW SKIN

The skin on your elbows gets wrinkly and saggy just like the skin on your knees. Your elbows take a beating throughout life, after all. Not only is the skin on your elbows being stretched every time you bend your elbow, it's also always rubbing against things like clothing. No wonder your skin on your elbow may grow a little thicker—it's just trying to protect itself. Not to mention, of course, that elbow skin is just naturally dryer than other skin on your body. The appearance of your elbows might bother you less than your knees, though—you can't see your elbows when you look in the mirror, plus you have less skin on your elbows than your knees, so the wrinkles and crinkles don't show as much.

Yet that doesn't mean you shouldn't show those elbows some love. Because elbow skin can also get dry from all the bending and moving you do in a day's time—not to mention the amount of time you spend propped up on your elbows—you should start giving it a little extra lubricant early, regardless of your age. One tried-and-true strategy? Coconut oil. Dab some on each elbow after you step out of the shower or before you head to bed.

LIGHTEN YOUR WORKLOAD

Being stressed at work, America's top stressor, could lead to exhaustion, which could accelerate your rate of biological aging. So see if you can cut your workload a little.

In a study from *PLOS One* of over 2,900 men and women aged thirty to sixty-four, those who had the most severe exhaustion and experienced high stress on a weekly basis had greater biological aging, shown through shorter telomeres (the caps at the ends of your DNA strands). Researchers suggest that chronic work stress may make your body age faster than it normally would. Work stress has also been linked to increased risk of heart issues like atrial fibrillation.

Although short periods of stress aren't damaging, chronic stress is, which is why you should monitor your well-being at work. If you're having problems sleeping or controlling your emotions or experiencing aches and pains for no reason, you might be taking on too much at work.

The best way to alleviate the problem is to somehow reduce your stress at work, either by reassigning some responsibilities or fixing a bad situation. If those solutions aren't feasible in the short term, at least take better care of yourself by logging the proper amount of sleep and following healthy lifestyle habits. Most importantly, allow time to recover each day from stress, which means not working after-hours at home, not accepting continuous overtime, and taking time for relaxation and social and physical activities.

If your entire job is really making you downright miserable, ask yourself if you really want to live this way every day. You could be jeopardizing your health in a serious way, so consider a job change if possible.

USE A HEADSET WHEN TALKING ON YOUR CELL PHONE

Your cell phone harbors ten times more bacteria than toilet seats, and every time you put that phone next to the skin on your face, those bacteria transfer over, mixing with the toxins, facial oils, and other irritants you collect on your face every day. That's why you might notice more acne on the side of your face where you hold the phone.

What's worse—the light from your screens could be making your skin produce more pigmentation, which could lead to premature age spots. If you're already dealing with melasma, a skin problem that causes brownish patches on the face (and forearms and neck), the phone's heat could increase the problem. The light from your cell phone could also damage collagen and lead to premature wrinkling.

So what's the best way to avoid this skin damage? Go hands-free by using a headset or earpiece whenever you're talking on your phone.

FILTER YOUR WATER

You might think your tap water is totally safe to drink. But here's what you may not know: tap water, even if your local authorities have deemed it safe, has to cross miles of pipes to reach your faucet, and along the way, it's picking up all sorts of particles, including industrial runoff, toxic by-products from manure and fertilizer, pesticides, and other unpleasant things.

Since 2010, the Environmental Working Group has been testing pollutants in tap water across America, and their findings aren't pretty: test results on over 48,000 water utilities in all fifty states between 2010 and 2015 found 267 contaminants. A whopping 93 percent of these contaminants have been linked with increased risk of cancer, and 78 percent have been linked with nervous system and brain damage. Other issues include problems with fertility, hormone disruption, and harm to developing children—even fetuses.

That's why you should install some type of water filtration system at home—even a filtering water pitcher or countertop system—and then fill reusable bottles to take with you. You can even buy inexpensive portable filters for reusable bottles in case you're in a pinch and can't access fresh water.

Another note: bottled water isn't any safer, as the Environmental Protection Agency even says that it's not safer than tap water. Plus, those plastic bottles will litter the earth.

SAY GOODBYE TO HEAVY EARRINGS

Gravity always wins, even when it comes to your ears. Sagging earlobes will make you look older, so it's time to start paying attention to those little flaps of skin.

First, put sunscreen on those earlobes when you apply it to your face and neck. You're probably getting more sun damage there than you realize, which can deteriorate skin health. More importantly, if you're wearing earrings, avoid long, heavy ones. The area of skin that holds them up is very small, and the weight of those earrings not only stretches those earring holes so they look more like slits but also drags your earlobes down, increasing the sagging effect and perhaps even making sagging permanent. If clip-on earrings are out of the question, stick with studs and light hoops. Damage already done? Talk with a dermatologist, who can recommend the appropriate solutions.

DARKEN YOUR BROWS

One trick to looking younger might lie in your brows. As you age, the color of your brows fades, which decreases your facial contrast. Yet studies show that the more facial contrast people have, the younger they look. In fact, in one study in which researchers showed pictures of two identical faces, one with more contrast and the other with less, people agreed that the face with more contrast looked younger than the face with low contrast almost 80 percent of the time.

That's where makeup can come in handy. You can use a brow pencil if you have one, but if not, you can also use a mascara brush in a pinch. First, wipe off excess mascara on the edge of the container. Then use a light touch when applying to the eyebrows so it doesn't appear *too* dark or smear. Because eyebrows aren't usually the same color as your hair, choose a brow pencil or mascara that's lighter than your hair; otherwise, if they're the same color or darker, they'll look unnatural.

DON'T YO-YO DIET

Constantly cycling your weight up and down isn't only bad for your health, it can also wreak havoc on your skin.

While crash diets can work in the short term, they do nothing to promote long-term weight-loss success, and in fact, they often do the exact opposite. You might initially lose the weight, but after the "crash" period is over and you go back to your regular diet, studies show that most people regain all the weight—and then some. That yo-yoing in weight can take a toll on the skin, causing it to stretch, sag, and wrinkle. Over time, your skin will look even older than your years as a result.

That's why it's time to steer clear of any crazy fad diets. So if you shouldn't diet, what should you do? Adopt a healthy, balanced lifestyle by eating more whole plant foods, which will naturally help you lose and keep it off long term.

EAT BREAKFAST

Mom was right: breakfast really is the most important meal of the day, helping you stay healthier in the long haul. Numerous studies have shown that eating breakfast is linked to a healthier weight, better cholesterol levels, and improved heart health.

Skipping breakfast has actually been linked to an increased risk of heart disease. One reason? A study from the *Journal of the American College of Cardiology* showed that breakfast skippers had more hardening of the arteries—a precursor for heart disease—than people who ate breakfast. Skippers also had the highest blood pressure, body mass index, waist circumference (they tend to not only eat more overall, but also nosh more unhealthy foods during the day), and blood lipids. Overall, they had an unhealthier lifestyle, as they were more likely to drink alcohol frequently, smoke, and eat a bad diet. Researchers suggest that lack of breakfast causes hormonal imbalances in the body and changes circadian rhythms.

If you're not used to eating breakfast, eat less before bed so you wake up hungrier, and start with small breakfasts as you adopt this new habit.

MAKE A FACE MASK FROM COFFEE GROUNDS

Did you know that using coffee grounds on your skin can help fight the effects of aging? Skincare products often use coffeeberry, harvesting it from the coffee plant's fruit. When used topically, coffeeberry has been shown to improve fine lines, pigmentation issues, wrinkles, and overall appearance. You can find it in skincare products, but if they are too expensive for your budget, put your used coffee grounds to work instead. Doing so has been shown in studies to decrease the effects of sun damage, reducing wrinkles, increasing the skin's thickness, and preventing water loss. Applying antioxidant-rich coffee grounds to your skin also stimulates blood flow, which brightens the skin.

For a simple mask, you'll need 1 tablespoon of your morning's coffee grounds, 2 tablespoons of ground oats, and 1 tablespoon of honey. Mix and apply to your face for twenty minutes. Rinse with warm water.

LOOK AT YOUR CEREAL'S NUTRITIONAL FACTS

Think your "healthy" cereal earns a dietitian's stamp of approval?

If you've chosen a cereal with whole grains, give yourself a pat on the back. That's at least a start. But what you may not realize is that many of these healthy-sounding cereals actually contain high amounts of added sugar. With sugar comes glucose spikes, and that spells wrinkles.

So do a little more sleuthing when it comes to those labels:

1. Look for a cereal that's almost entirely (or all) whole grain. The first ingredient should be bran or whole grain. Another clue? The label should say "100 percent whole grain."
2. Now check the sugars (a new food label is out that shows the amount of *added* sugars on packaging) and choose cereals with no more than a total of 7 grams of sugar for lower-calorie cereals, 11 grams for higher-calorie cereals.
3. Check serving size, too, to see how many calories you'll be chomping.
4. Make sure it contains unprocessed fiber (oats, whole-grain wheat, and wheat bran are good choices).
5. Find a cereal with under 2.5 grams of saturated fat, according to the Center for Science in the Public Interest.

TAN WITH TURMERIC

Getting a sun-kissed look can be key in feeling—and some might argue, looking—younger. How can you do it sans the harmful rays of the sun? Turn to turmeric.

As you learned in hack #72, you can use sunless tanners, but they're not always as easy to use, and they can irritate some people's skin. So reach for more natural products like turmeric, which can give that skin a radiant glow and a bit of color.

You'll need 1 cup of organic coconut oil (keep it in its original state) and 3 tablespoons of powdered turmeric. Slather it on your skin twice daily as you would any cream or lotion, letting it sit for a few minutes, and then rinse it off so that it doesn't stain your clothes. Store any leftovers of the mixture in a cool, dark place.

STAND UP

Too much sedentary time is bad for your health and your longevity. Here's an easy way to combat that: stand up when you're waiting for something. Think about all the waiting you do in life: waiting to see a doctor, waiting to board a plane, waiting for a table at a restaurant, and so on.

Now think about what you're doing as you wait. If you're like most people, you're probably looking for a chair. No more. Instead, use that time to stand—or even better, move around. Standing, after all, burns fifty more calories an hour than sitting—do this for thirty extra minutes a day and you could actually lose a little over 5 pounds in a year without changing anything else. You'll get even more benefits if you can move around during this time—walk around the airport terminal, doctor's office, or restaurant grounds.

MOISTURIZE MORE OFTEN WHEN YOU'RE ON MEDICATIONS

Anything you put in your mouth, including medications, can affect your skin, which is why you should amp up your skincare routine if you're on a medication.

Certain medications, like nonsteroidal anti-inflammatory drugs, antibiotics, and diuretics, can cause photosensitivity, which means that your skin will be more sensitive to the sun and could become damaged (read: wrinkles and pigmentation changes) more easily. Meanwhile, other medications like corticosteroids can lower your body's supply of collagen and elastin.

While you shouldn't stop taking these medications, do check with your doctor to find out how any medications you're taking could affect your skin. Then make skincare a bigger priority. Make sure you're using sunscreen daily and reapplying it frequently throughout the day. Also, use a retinol cream at night to help stimulate your skin's production of collagen.

ENJOY DARK CHOCOLATE IN THE MORNING

Here's the best Rx for better, younger-looking skin: eat a piece of dark chocolate every day, preferably in the morning. Chocolate's long been heralded for its benefits on brain and heart health, but some research also points to it as a natural sunscreen of sorts (sorry, you still need sunscreen, though). According to one study from the *Journal of Cosmetic Dermatology*, the anti-inflammatory and antioxidant activity of the flavonols in 20 grams of dark chocolate a day helped reduce the risk of sunburn, essentially lowering sensitivity to the sun among the dark chocolate eaters.

High-antioxidant chocolate may also improve skin elasticity or suppleness, skin thickness, hydration, and microcirculation, all of which improve your skin's appearance.

When choosing the best chocolate, look for one that contains at least 70 percent cocoa—milk chocolate doesn't cut it—and the fewest ingredients possible. And remember that although chocolate is considered a superfood, noted for its benefits on the heart and brain, it still comes with calories, so indulge in small amounts. Some experts recommend choosing cocoa powder, as it contains the most flavonols but the least amount of calories. Better yet, nosh that chocolate in the morning, as studies have found that this timing can aid weight loss and boost brain function.

BOOST YOUR INTAKE OF OMEGA-3S

Fat is your skin's friend, which is why you want to make sure you're getting your fill of those healthy omega-3 fatty acids. Without enough healthy fat in your body, your skin will be more prone to drying. Yet by getting the right fat, namely alpha-linolenic acid (ALA, which you can get from plant-based sources of omega-3 fatty acids), you'll be able to fight age-related skin dryness. Even better? Your skin's elasticity can be improved by eating more omega-3 fatty acids, which include not only ALA but also docosahexaenoic acid (DHA) and eicosapentaenoic acid (EPA).

Your heart will also benefit, as studies show that omega-3 fatty acids can lower inflammation, blood pressure, and cholesterol and may prevent plaque from building in your arteries.

You can get omega-3 fatty acids from fish (see hack #74 for more information about the best fish choices and how they can help your heart) or plant-based sources like chia seeds, flaxseed, and walnuts. If you're following a vegan diet, know that you may not get enough DHA and EPA from plants alone, so you may have to supplement. Look for vegan versions with algae-based sources.

VENTILATE YOUR HOUSE

The air you breathe in your house really affects your health. The air inside your house or apartment is equally as important as, if not more important than, outdoor air pollution. Estimates indicate that people spend 90 percent of their time indoors, and that indoor air could be up to five times more polluted than outdoor air!

In the short term, you might experience issues like dizziness; headaches; irritation of your eyes, nose, and throat; and even fatigue. In the long run, bad indoor air quality could lead to heart disease, respiratory illnesses, and cancer, all of which could be fatal. And yes, like outdoor pollution, indoor air pollution can affect skin aging, especially if you live with a smoker or you smoke.

So how do you know if your indoor air quality is an issue? Simple: see if any symptoms you're experiencing disappear when you leave your house for a few days. If those symptoms return when you come home, you know you've got a problem. You can also have your indoor air quality tested. You can buy a home air quality test, use an indoor air quality monitor like Speck, or ask your heating and air conditioning company if they do air quality checks.

To keep indoor air clean, open windows and doors when the weather allows so your house airs out, especially when you're doing things like painting or sanding. You should also:

- Run window or attic fans or a window air conditioner that's set with the vent control open.
- Set up bathroom and kitchen fans so they exhaust outdoors.
- Turn on the exhaust fan above your stove when cooking.

If you have a smoker in the house, refer to hack #30 for specific tips on clearing the air.

GIVE YOURSELF AN AT-HOME FACIAL STEAM

There's a reason many professional facials include a steam: it helps increase your skin's oil production, which not only moisturizes your skin but also gives you a youthful glow. The one caveat? If you have rosacea or are susceptible to acne, you should probably avoid the heat.

You don't need to wait for a professional to do it for you, though. It's simple to do a facial steam at home. Just boil 1 to 2 quarts of water and pour it into a glass bowl. You can even add a few drops of your favorite essential oil if you like. Mix the oils in (or not) and then let the water sit for several minutes until its steam is warm but not hot. Hold your head about 6 to 8 inches from the water and place a towel over your head, tenting it so you trap the steam. Stay here for up to ten minutes before rinsing your face with cool water and then moisturizing.

DON'T SKIP MEALS

If you're a regular meal skipper, watch out: you could be prematurely aging your skin without even knowing it. Whether you forget or just don't have time to eat, skipping meals isn't a good idea (and if you're doing it to lose weight, think again, as starvation diets lead to negative health consequences and even more weight gain once you go off the diet). As obvious as this sounds, not only will your body not get the fuel it needs, your skin also won't get the nutrients it needs, making it age faster. Skipping meals could also lead to more dehydrated skin, making those wrinkles and fine lines more visible. Plus, when you skip meals, you're more likely to be so hungry later that you veer toward unhealthy grub or you overeat, which can also lead to skin issues. One study found that when people skipped meals, they bought 31 percent more junk food at the store in a hungry state versus when they'd eaten a snack before shopping. And no food means no energy to exercise, so clearly skipping meals is just a terrible idea all around.

Bottom line? Plan every meal, perhaps scheduling your meal times in your calendar every night before you go to bed. Don't go to the grocery store when you're starving so you're more likely to make positive choices. Then set alarms to remind you to eat. If the time for food prep is the issue, try doing all of your week's food prep on your quietest day.

MOISTURIZE WITH OLIVE OIL IN A PINCH

Out of moisturizer? Olive oil to the rescue!

This kitchen staple has been used for skin health for centuries—and for good reason. It's loaded with antioxidants and squalene, a natural moisturizer, both of which can help aging skin. Olive oil not only hydrates the skin but also softens fine lines and wrinkles.

Fortunately, olive oil absorbs well, but your skin will absorb it even better after a shower. You can use it on your whole body, even your face.

A bonus idea? Pat a little olive oil on that face when you need a quick freshener before an event. The oil will add a natural glow to your skin.

EAT SOME SEAWEED

Seaweed in your salad might not sound appetizing—until you realize that seaweed is a superfood for your skin. Seaweed is loaded with essential minerals like copper, iron, and magnesium, all of which can improve your skin, nails, and hair. That's one reason it's been added to skincare products, but you should also add seaweed to your diet to get even more benefits. Not only can seaweed slow the aging process inside, it can also add protection from pollutants to the skin, give nails some strength, and add shine to hair.

There are numerous seaweeds you can find at the grocery store, including hijiki, wakame, nori (which you'll find in sushi rolls), kombu, and kelp noodles. Depending on the type of seaweed, you can add it to salad, stir-fry, vegetables, and noodle dishes. You might even try some of the dried seaweed snacks that are popping up on grocery store shelves. They give you a healthy dose of the nutrients seaweed is famous for, including iodine and vitamins A, C, and B_{12} (which is beneficial if you're a vegan and looking for a non-animal source of this vitamin), and they're great if you're craving a low-calorie, salty treat. The one caveat? If you have any thyroid issues, the high iodine content of seaweed may make it risky for you to eat, so ask your doctor first.

CELEBRATE YOUR AGE

It's time to stop complaining about getting older and instead celebrate your age!

Granted, it's not always fun to see your hair go gray or your skin get more wrinkly. But age really is just a number, and if you don't mind, it doesn't matter. Only you can decide what that number means, and know that age doesn't have to define you. Just look to the former president George H.W. Bush, who went skydiving on his ninetieth birthday.

So view each birthday as a celebration and find a way to honor the years you've spent on this earth—and all the years you have yet to enjoy. Maybe you donate your age in dollars to your favorite non-profit organization, walk your age in miles over a certain period (for instance, if you're turning 50, you could set a goal to walk 5 miles a day for ten days), spend a month doing as many random acts of kindness as your age, dedicate your age in minutes to doing something you love doing (and rarely make time to do) on your birthday, or treat yourself to a special birthday gift equal to your age in dollars (talk about something to look forward to each year!). The simple fact is that it's a gift to be alive, so enjoy the present!

IMPROVE YOUR LIFE—
One Hack at a Time!

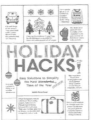

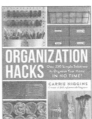

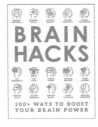

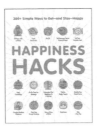

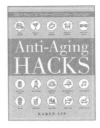

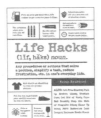

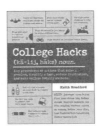

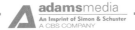

adamsmedia
An Imprint of Simon & Schuster
A CBS COMPANY